MITES NO MORE

How To Get Rid of Bird Mites and Other Crawling, Biting Parasites Forever

---

Robert E. Johnson

Mites No More
Copyright © 2017 by Harmony House

All rights reserved. No part of this book may be reproduced or transmitted, in whole or in part, in any form or by any means electronic or mechanical, including photocopying, recording, or by any information storage and retrieval system now known or hereafter invented, without written permission from the publisher.

Paperback edition

ISBN 978-0-9640347-4-7

Published by Harmony House
2516 Waukegan Road, Suite 301
Glenview, IL 60025

The author and publisher make no warranties, expressed or implied, with respect to the information contained herein. The author is not engaged in rendering legal, financial, medical or other professional services. If the reader requires professional advice of any kind, he or she is urged to seek it directly from a competent professional. Resources mentioned in this book are for information only, and the author and publisher shall not be held liable for any damages whatsoever in connection with, or arising out of, the reader's use of them.

Contents

Introduction 5
Chapter 1 Get Inspired 14
Chapter 2 Learn the Lessons 23
Chapter 3 Begin the Battle 27
Chapter 4 Know the Enemy 41
Chapter 5 Attack the Mites 49
Chapter 6 Clean and Seal 55
Chapter 7 Set Routines 69
Chapter 8 Do the Laundry 79
Chapter 9 Get to Bed 87
Chapter 10 Repel the Mites 95
Chapter 11 Host No More 105
Chapter 12 Eliminate Them All 117
Appendix 127

Introduction

You're about to read a scary story. But unlike the tall tales told in books and movies, this frightening story is completely true.

Luckily, there is a positive ending to our story. But it took us a long time to get there. If you're reading this, you're probably wondering how to end a mite infestation. You will find the solution in the pages of this book.

Of course, a mite problem isn't fatal. But a serious bird mite infestation can still be a nightmare, as ours was.

Imagine yourself laying in bed at night. You feel your body swarming with tiny, crawling insects. They are moving all over you, actively crawling on every inch of your skin. Some are biting you.

These are extremely tiny creatures, virtually invisible to the eye. Though you can't see them, you definitely feel them as they crawl on you. And they're not just roaming over your skin. Some are biting, too. Their bites are sometimes sharp and sudden, like a needle jabbing you.

The tiny insects may also crawl into the openings of your body. Not just your eyes, nose and mouth -- but *every* opening. And they bite you in those area, too. Ouch! No, bird mites won't kill you. But the relentless torture is absolutely awful.

During the day, the problem continues. Some areas of your home may have greater or lesser infestation. You avoid the "hot spots" as best you can. But the creatures can sense where you are. If you move to a less active room, they soon find you there. You may feel them jumping onto your legs from the floor, or dropping down on to your head and neck from the ceiling.

If your home is badly infested, your vehicle easily becomes infested too. Since mites are on your body and clothes, some easily transfer to your car. They may also settle into your workspace. For example, they may hide in the crevices of your office chair.

Night after night and day after day, an unrecognized mite problem can rapidly compound itself. Unless you take quick steps to deal with the problem, it can quickly reach a point where painful bites are almost continuous, as happened to us.

At that crisis level, we desperately tried everything: pesticides and professional exterminators, strenuous house cleaning, body purification, medical remedies, and everything else we could think of. Most of it had limited results. While a few remedies had some effect, each time the mites adapted, and came back stronger than before. It wasn't until we stumbled upon the right combination of steps that we were able to finally solve the problem completely.

End of the Nightmare

This book was written to help you *totally eliminate* the bird mites (or other tiny, unidentified parasites) that crawl on your skin and bite you. If you or your loved ones are suffering from an invasion of these obnoxious pests, you're not alone. From our research and outreach, we believe that parasitic bird mites (fowl mites, northern avian mites, and tropical bird mites) are a growing problem for humans, afflicting many thousands of households.

Please understand that if you have an infestation of bedbugs, fleas, or other non-mite creatures, or if you suffer from Morgellons disease, these strategies may not apply. Our main focus here is the eradication of bird mites. You first become aware of these extremely tiny (virtually invisible) bugs when you feel them crawling on your skin and biting you.

Sadly, the problem is often misunderstood or dismissed by professionals, including many in the medical community. Mite sufferers are left with no recourse but to find solutions on their own.

MITES NO MORE was written by a former bird mite sufferer, now 100% mite free for the past seven years. By following the advice in these pages, you too can achieve complete victory in your battle against parasitic bird mites.

We Tried Everything

Every possible remedy we heard about or dreamed up, we tried. Despite our positive attitude, most of the tactics let us down. There were many crushed hopes along the way. Sometimes, a new approach would seem to be working. Then, just a day or two later, the mites would be back, as aggressive as ever.

During the ordeal, we spent money on many things that didn't work. We devoted many waking hours each day to fighting the bugs. And the restless few hours of sleep we managed to get at night were usually uncomfortable, as bird mites are more active at night.

As you will read, some of our ideas may seem crazy. We doubt you'll read about those ideas anywhere but in this book. We'll also share the effective anti-mite tricks we learned from others.

In trying so many things, we figured, what did we have to lose?

All of the trial and error, plus our stubborn refusal to quit, finally led us to the right combination of strategies. The result was eventual, final and total *mite elimination.*

No, all the bird mites didn't vanish instantly, on one magical day. That would have been nice. But they did gradually begin to die off over the course of about a month or two -- once we stumbled upon the right set of strategies. Best of all they have not returned, and it has been seven years as of this writing. Today, we remain 100% mite free. Our home, vehicle, wardrobe and workplace are once again as they used to be – totally mite free.

We consider this a true blessing, one that we will never take for granted. One benefit from the ordeal: we can better appreciate many of the little blessings in life, such as a good night's sleep, more than ever.

During many long days and nights, we never lost hope. Two sayings come to mind here:

- "God never gives us anything we can't handle"
- "That which does not kill us, makes us stronger"

The strategies we followed and the products we used are described in the pages ahead. We sincerely hope our detailed instructions help to eliminate your mite problem completely.

The Web as a Resource

Thank goodness for the Internet. If not for the support and information we found online, we would have been in total despair over the devastating situation.

We recall late one night, in our endless web search for clues, coming upon someone's description of a serious mite infestation. The anonymous post described it as

"Living in Dante's seventh circle of hell". That is about as accurate a description as any!

Just knowing we weren't alone was a comfort. If you've felt totally isolated because of a mite infestation, please know that others are struggling with the same situation. You are not alone! And you must keep fighting, even if things appear hopeless right now. You CAN overcome a mite problem and return to a normal life. We are living proof of that.

Watch Out for Faulty Advice

While the Internet was helpful, we quickly learned that there is plenty of bad information out there about eradicating tiny biting bugs. This is especially true regarding bird mite infestations of humans.

There are quite a few websites on this topic. Only a few have worthwhile tips. And while message boards were not very helpful, they did offer a sense of community with fellow sufferers.

Unfortunately, most websites repeat the same faulty info, over and over again. These sites seem to exist only to make money for someone. It's doubtful these site owners ever had personal experience with bird mites. The sites are full of copied or made-up information, apparently to sell products or to get paid clicks.

Don't let the Internet distract you from learning proven mite elimination steps. We suggest you visit the web later, AFTER you finish reading the helpful pages ahead.

NOTE: If you wish to jump directly to specific mite elimination tactics, begin with Chapter 5. Chapters 1-4 contain helpful information and inspiration, so we strongly recommend you read those chapters too.

Chapter One: GET INSPIRED

Begin each day with a positive mindset. This is probably the most important ingredient for total eradication of a mite population in your home.

As we mentioned in the introduction, even in the darkest hours we always clung to the belief that one day, we would be completely free of the tiny biting and crawling pests.

We always expected to achieve eventual victory, despite the fact that bird mites are the most persistent, seemingly indestructible creatures we'd ever encountered. Thanks to our ever-optimistic outlook, we refused to accept any attitude of defeat. We constantly visualized a positive outcome.

Reasons for Optimism

For those who think that a good attitude is a worthless waste of time and energy, here are two practical reasons to be optimistic. A positive attitude helps your mind stay open to new ways of problem solving. And it helps you to stay in action, despite the setbacks. A negative attitude has the opposite effect.

Negativity makes every effort feel hopeless from the start. It discourages you from making a full force attack, which limits your results.

While online, we discovered a loose community of mite sufferers. They seemed to hang out at the same few message boards, looking for bits of information, hope or companionship they may find. Every rumor or insight gets discussed at length.

In our search for a cure, we read through hundreds upon hundreds of these posts. The messages from these intrepid warriors were sometimes stark and depressing. Other posts were heartwarming. Despite the limited good news anyone had to share, many sufferers displayed a caring attitude toward others who were in worse shape.

In retrospect, after reading all those unhappy messages, it's surprising that we stayed optimistic. Here's why we say that.

In all the many long nights we spent reading those messages, we never came across a single report from <u>anyone</u> who said they were completely cured of mites. Just the opposite, in fact.

We recall one sad person who posted a message saying they'd been fighting mites for over a decade, and had exhausted both their funds and their health. Not exactly uplifting to read that! Another woman was living out of a suitcase, traveling constantly from hotel to hotel, trying to outrun the mites, but never quite doing it. Another hopeless situation.

There were a handful of reports from people who "had heard of somebody" who had a 100% cure, but details were vague as to how they did it. Few hard facts were ever presented about those miracle cures.

A few CLAIMED to have eliminated mites by dubious means, such as spraying Windex everywhere in their house. We can easily dismiss those reports, based on our own direct experience. We actually tried nearly everything we heard about online. Trust us -- Windex does *not* eliminate mites (water is the number one ingredient in Windex, so spraying it around will actually worsen a mite problem).

The Good News

There is good news in all of this. There are definite, proven ways to eliminate bird mites. Follow our guidelines, and we believe that in a relatively short time the mites will be far less of a nuisance for you, and eventually you will rid yourself completely of mites, and restore your life's balance to what it used to be. Yes, it is a rigorous program to follow. We don't claim it will be effortless. But the results will be worth it.

 As we mentioned in the Introduction, a few of our suggestions may cause you to say "Oh, I could never do THAT. What would people think?"

Well, please discard that limited thinking! You must do whatever is required, simply because that's how you solve a bird mite infestation once and for all.

The Mental Attitude You Need

Here is the mental attitude to develop right now. Think of yourself as a *warrior*. You are a very determined fighter who will not quit until victory is yours.

In a military boot camp, this same kind of attitude is instilled in recruits. It becomes an integral part of their thinking. With this attitude, along with proper training, new soldiers soon learn that they're capable of doing things they never imagined were possible.

The fact is, YOU are capable of doing things you never imagined possible. And if you are ready and willing to make some real changes, and let go of limited thinking and worry about what others may think, you're well on the way to resolving the infestation once and for all.

Let's consider the insect enemy you're facing. Have you been building up this army of mites in your mind, as something powerful, something invincible, something to be feared? Do you wish you could just run away and hide from them somehow, find a way to escape?

To be blunt, forget that crap! You need to adopt a reckless, cocky, unshakable warrior attitude. You are going to face down the enemy and defeat them completely. Know with certainty that you will be the ultimate winner, when the last battle is over and the war is done.

Compare Us Against Them

Let's take stock of both sides in this battle. How do the good guys (humans) line up against the seemingly invincible bird mite army? Which side in this war has the ultimate winning edge -- our side, or the enemy side?

Bird mites have the following advantages:

- Size – mites can easily hide and are very difficult for humans to see
- Rapid reproduction – a few mites can quickly become many mites
- Resistance - mites aren't stopped by pesticides (see appendix notes)
- Adaptability – bird mites can adapt fast to many anti-mite strategies
- Nocturnal – bird mites get more active when humans sleep
- Survivability – bird mites can live 90 days (or more) away from a host
- Evolutionary history – mites have been on Earth longer than humans

Clearly, a bird mite infestation means you face a formidable foe. But never surrender. Consider the major advantages that the humans have in this conflict.

Humans have the following advantages over mites:

- Vastly superior intelligence – we reason, we will, we act decisively
- Quick adaptation – we can rapidly change many variables
- Speed & Distance - we can move farther and faster than mites
- Weapons arsenal – our tools of war go way beyond pesticides
- Shared tactics - we can learn mite-killing secrets from others
- Environment - we can control and modify our indoor environment

Yes, humans can defeat the worst mite infestations.

Bottom line: superior intelligence, speed, tactical knowledge, vast array of weapons and basic persistence means that the *humans have the winning advantage*. Never, ever doubt it!

As you read this book, you may notice we sometimes use military terms to describe the battle against mites. We're not war mongers, nor are we former military. We do have great respect for those who protect and defend our nation.

In taking on a warrior mindset, we decided to adopt the same fighting attitude that we admire in the valiant members of the military. That tough-minded, resilient attitude has helped win major wars, and likewise it can help you avoid defeatism and keep you moving forward. It can help you -- IF you're willing to adopt it.

Stages of Acceptance

We hope you'll be tough minded. But that's not to say some emotions may surface. It's good to be aware of these emotional stages. Here are some you might experience.

DISBELIEF -- The mind-numbing extent of your dilemma is staring you in the face, but you cannot accept the reality of the situation. You refuse to believe it's actually happening. You might try to ignore it, which isn't smart. The easiest time to get rid of mites is before they're fully established in your home.

SADNESS – Once the cold hard facts of the mite infestation finally hit you, you may start feeling sorry for yourself. Tears may flow, you might feel emotionally distraught and overwhelmed at the burden you feel. You grieve over the loss of your previous lifestyle, or at the solitary nature of your condition. Sad feelings might hit you unexpectedly during the day or late at night when you're alone with your thoughts.

ANGER — Once the sadness starts to fade, angry feelings may surface. For example, if you suspect that someone else caused your mite problem, your anger might be directed toward them. Or your angry feelings might even be toward God, the universe, or fate. You might even ask yourself emotional questions such as "Why the hell did this happen to me? What did I ever do to deserve this?" (Cursing and swearing are optional here)

ACCEPTANCE—This is when you finally set aside negative emotions, and accept the fact that like it or not, you are in a real battle.

This stage is when you can best put on the psychological armor and the attitude of a true warrior, and visualize and develop the powerful inner belief that you will achieve eventual victory. It's not just possible, it's inevitable!

Picture a Motivating, Positive End Result

We suggest that today, you begin visualizing something meaningful that you will experience, once you have defeated the bird mites and the problem has been fully resolved. For example, you might visualize a very special celebration you will have by yourself or with your loved ones. Of course, no one but you needs to know the actual reason for the celebration, unless you wish to share it with them.

In our case, we visualized the creation of this book, and how it might help others who were fighting bird mites. We kept this meaningful goal in mind. It not only helped us work harder to solve our mite problem, but it also helped us maintain an "up" attitude.

We recall hearing a story long ago, about a man who was imprisoned in a concentration camp during World War II. There was almost no food to eat. Most of the prisoners were malnourished and sick. Despite his personal hunger, this man decided he'd share his daily food ration with others who most needed it. Though many of the other prisoners eventually died of starvation and illness, the sharing man was able to survive in decent health. He later credited his attitude of helping others with keeping him strong.

Likewise, we suggest you think about something significant and positive that you will do, once you're past this temporary annoying problem. Hold this thought in your mind to boost your spirits, fuel your determination, and keep yourself in a more positive state of mind. Sighing, crying, and a few swear words are to be expected. But please get past the emotional baggage as quickly as you can. Refuse to accept the victim mentality.

Lastly, please remember that while you are suffering with a horrible mite infestation, there are countless others around the world in hospital beds or on battlefields, suffering far worse fates than your own.

Chapter Two: LEARN THE LESSONS

While the mite infestation was happening to us, we tried to view the experience as a trial by fire, one that we would eventually overcome. In other words, we looked at it as some sort of cosmic test that we needed to pass, so we could get on with life.

During the daily tests we faced, we tried to see what lessons we were supposed to learn from them. We kept a journal to track our progress. Being spiritual, we also leaned on God and prayers for support. We also made prayer requests of religious groups (these can often be made online, anonymously).

Please don't dismiss the spiritual strategy. There have been numerous studies of the power of prayer. Anyone who is fighting against bird mites can use all the help they can get.

Lifestyle Changes

One thing that you will quickly find with a mite problem is that many of your old, comfortable lifestyle routines get totally disrupted. You quickly learn that you can no longer just come home, flop down on the couch, open a beer or other beverage, and watch TV for hours on end. Nor can you slump in a chair, surf the web, or play video games all day or night. The mites will soon find you, they start crawling and biting, and you are compelled to do something about it. You may also pass up invitations to socialize, to avoid spreading the problem to others.

It's a natural reaction to mourn the loss of those old routines. You may feel those activities were the "comfort food" that made life worth living -- but now, your moments of relaxation and escape have been stolen away by the nasty mite invasion.

At first, that's exactly how we felt about it.

Same Old Routines

But after giving it some thought, we realized that over a period of time, our life had gradually fallen into a series of stale routines. In fact, life had become nothing but one established routine, after another, after another.

Most people's lives tend to fall into this pattern. We wake up at about the same time each day. We dress in basically the same sets of clothes, we eat the same basic foods, we drive to the same places, we shop at the same stores.

In our off-hours at home, we amuse ourselves with the same sort of entertainment, over and over again. Perhaps we socialize with the same people, doing the same sorts of activities, again and again. Then we go to bed at about the same time. The next day, we wake up and do it all over again.

This can go on for years or even decades. For some, it may go on for the rest of their lives -- unless something comes along to blast us out of our dull routines, forcing us to adopt new patterns of living

After realizing the mite infestation had shattered all our comfortable old routines, we wondered if the crisis was actually the universe telling us it was time to make some changes to our old routines. Looking back, we are convinced of it.

Making Real Changes

The process of winning our mite battle forced us to make many changes. Some felt awkward or uncomfortable at first. But today we are in a far better place in every way. Had we not gone through that hellish experience, we can't imagine anything changing us in so many ways, other than perhaps a major medical crisis or a tragic accident.

So don't be afraid to let go of your old routines. It may be a bit stressful at first. You may resent the fact that you can't just go home and vegetate by the boob tube or spend hours on social media, as we once did. You may miss hanging out with friends, out of fear of spreading the bugs to others. You may not like having to change your usual diet (yes, that may be necessary), or change the clothes you wear, or alter your hygiene routine.

But anyone can be very adaptable, when we have to be. And if you are *truly committed* to ridding yourself of mites forever, then the lifestyle changes outlined here shouldn't be so difficult.

Chapter Three: BEGIN THE BATTLE

This is the story of how our bird mite infestation first began and how it unfolded. We'll include details about so-called professionals that we contacted for assistance, as well as our own attempts to battle the mites. We think you may find value in these details.

It all began on a summer afternoon as we were doing some routine chores outside our home. We noticed a large robin standing on a patch of lawn. What struck us was how odd this bird looked, as if it had some unusual problem.

The bird's feathers were askew and it had a weird, crazed appearance. Unlike a typical wild bird, the robin completely ignored us, even though we were standing just a few feet away.

What happened next was even more surprising. The bird marched right past us. It kept going on a beeline toward our ranch-style home. The robin hopped up the step to the front porch. Then, inches from the closed front door, it slowly leaned forward and rested its head on the cement stoop.

Obviously the creature was not well. But we hoped that after a short rest, it might revive and fly away. So we let it stay where it was, thinking that was the humane thing to do. We didn't realize the bird was in the process of dying.

Months later, we'd think back to the events of that day. Would things have turned out differently, had we immediately chased that unhealthy robin away? But at the time, we were being kind by letting it stay by the door and rest for a while.

As the afternoon progressed, we quietly went in and out the door several times. Each time, we stepped past the bird which was visibly breathing but barely moving. That evening, we went outside again. Now it was clear that the bird was dead. Using a shovel, we picked up the carcass and carried it to a wooded area some distance away. We tossed the dead robin into the undergrowth.

From Bird Host to Human Host

We later learned about documented cases of bird mites transferring from bird hosts to human hosts, when the bird host is no longer available (see appendix). Commonly, this happens when a bird abandons a nest that is loaded with mites. If the nest is anywhere near a house (such as on a window sill, roof, air conditioner unit, or nearby tree), the abandoned bird mites may enter the home seeking a new host.

In our case, we believe the dying robin was badly infested with bird mites. Perhaps the parasites had taken such a toll, they had caused the weakened bird to succumb. When it died, our home was the closest target. Thus, I became the next victim of those bird mites.

Unfortunately, textbooks at medical schools still teach that while bird mites might randomly bite a human for a day or maybe a week, they never latch onto humans over the long term.

Well, if that concept was ever true, it clearly is no longer accurate. There are in fact documented cases of humans being severely infested with mites for long periods of time. An etymologist (insect expert) at a major university has stated that he has observed such cases (see appendix).

Perhaps when the medical textbooks were written, bird mites did not accept humans as long term hosts. But these tiny creatures reproduce quickly AND can evolve rapidly, in order to survive.

Another factor to consider is that many birds fly south for the winter. Possibly, some may become infested with *tropical* bird mites while wintering in southern climates.

Also, as with other creatures native to other lands, *tropical* mites may behave quite differently from domestic species like the northern avian mite. For example, compare the differences between native honeybees and Africanized bees, and between native ants and fire ants from south of the border. It's easy to imagine that tropical bird mites may be more aggressive and resilient than northern avian mites, which are commonly encountered in a henhouse or in the typical suburban setting.

Preying on human victims may simply be another path of survival for all bird mites, in an increasingly urbanized world.

Signs of Change

Returning to our story, it's now the evening of the day the robin died. We don't recall anything unusual happening that first night, but we do remember wondering about the strange death of the bird, right by our front door.

That night, we decided to jot down a few lines about it in a journal. In writing about the strange event, we wondered if it might be a harbinger of the future. Our optimistic little note said, 'Maybe this is a sign of a big change coming! ' That was an understatement, for sure.

Within a few days, we began to realize something unusual was happening. We began to feel hard bites on our skin. Were they mosquito bites? After all, it was the middle of summer. If so, how did so many mosquitoes get in the house? We made no connection at all between the bites and the bird that had died.

Those hard bites soon became more of a regular thing, especially in bed at night. Our legs and torso were the usual targets. The bites would sometimes swell and itch afterwards.

It became clear that bites were not from flying insects. There was no sign of them. Perhaps they were spider bites – although there was no sign of spiders, either. We went to a sporting goods store to buy a mosquito net. With that over the bed, we figured it would keep bugs away while we slept. We also sprayed the mattress and box spring with a household aerosol pesticide.
Despite those efforts, that night the bites were worse than ever. Had we somehow antagonized whatever was biting us? (Later we learned that bug spray does have that effect. Mites are mostly immune to pesticides, and the added moisture boosts their activity).

More and More Bites

Things began to get worse. The bites were multiplying and we broke out in a rash. There was temporary relief from bites when bathing or showering, but when stepping out of the shower, we'd literally feel things jumping onto us -- but we couldn't see the creatures, whatever they were. It was becoming a nightmarish situation.

By now, we were getting bites in the car and at the office. The worst place was at home. We felt crawling sensations most of the time. The bedroom had become a 'hot zone' and was now completely off limits. We couldn't be in that room for more than a few moments without multiple hard bites. The carpet and bed were fully infested.

So we tried sleeping on a plastic air mattress in another room, but soon the relentless, invisible bugs would find us. We were now getting hard bites everywhere. It was maddening, to say the least.

Because of our ignorance, initial apathy, and inability to fight whatever was attacking us, we gave the aggressive mite population enough time to explode. Since we were the one and only target, at this point life quickly became a living hell.

Identifying The Problem

Thankfully, once we began to do some research, the Internet quickly helped us identify just what sort of pest we were dealing with: *bird mites*. We remembered the dead robin. Now we made the connection.

As mentioned earlier, only a few websites were truly helpful. Those offered detailed suggestions, which we began to follow. We'll share the strategies that provided some relief.

Early on, we tried insect "bombs" which fog every room with pesticide. (You set off the aerosol bomb, quickly leave for a few hours, then return and open a window to air things out.) But the bombs were worthless and had zero effect. The mites were just as relentless as before! They are apparently fully resistant to pyretherin-based pesticides. That was one of the first disappointments.

Next we tried several flea pesticides. They had zero effect, other than apparently irritating the mites. The biting got worse. Obviously, fleas were not the problem.

We also tried various household bug sprays. None of them did anything, as the mites are resistant to all of them. We even tried a professional broad spectrum pesticide containing byrithrin, but it didn't help either. Nor did Sevin, or insecticide dusting powders.

Would a professional exterminator would be able to solve the crisis? Perhaps they'd have access to some little-known mite killing secrets.

Seeking Professional Help

We quickly phoned a number of pest control companies. No one we called would respond to a bird mite problem. All the outfits we called said they didn't handle mites. After still one more turn down, we begged the sympathetic manager to send over a serviceman, anyway. When he arrived, he was carrying a small tank sprayer but told us he had no idea if his stuff would kill mites or not. As we explained the extent of problem, and he realized how bad it was, he began to act skittish. We sensed that he wanted to leave before any mites jumped on him too.

He doubtfully asked if we had a sample of bird mites. He wanted to take it back to the shop and put it under the microscope. He said they like to see exactly what they're fighting, so they can see about exterminating them.

Having already read that pest companies like to get a sample, we'd purchased some adhesive bug traps. We'd placed these under a heat lamp in the living room to attract some mites. Sure enough, the trap soon had several tiny black specks stuck on the sticky surface. The pest guy was surprised that we had a sample to give him. He grabbed it, said someone would call to follow up, and hurried out the door.

When we later phoned the office for an update, the manager told us their office microscope wasn't strong enough to identify anything. So he'd mailed our sample to an expert. We called again a few days later, and he sheepishly said our sample was lost in shipping. Was this just a line, or the truth? The manager seemed very disinterested at this point. Maybe he thought we were imagining things. Obviously, this was getting us nowhere. We were back to square one.

We didn't know at that point if there was such a thing as a specialist in mite control or how to even find such a person, if one existed. The magnitude of the problem was beginning to dawn on us. How could we ever get rid of the bird mites?

Whole House Tenting

As we searched the Internet, we learned that an entire house can be completely covered and tented in plastic, and a powerful bug-killing gas is pumped inside the house where it remains for several days. (If you live in the Southern US or West coast, where termites are common, you may already be familiar with this concept.)

Deadly Vikane gas permeates every particle of a home, even inside the walls and timbers, eradicating every living thing. After the gas does its work, the tent is removed and the lighter-than-air gas floats away.

Sunlight breaks down the gas fumes to make them harmless and inert. The gas leaves the home safe to use, the furnishings in perfect condition, and the bugs dead. This sounded like the ideal solution to our problem.

Unfortunately, after again calling every local pest control company, they all told us that whole house tenting "just isn't done in this region". Apparently, the procedure is uncommon or completely unheard of in northern US states (where we lived).

If you happen to live in a region where whole house tenting is commonly accepted, such as the deep South or coastal California, perhaps Vikane gas will rid your home of mites. But it wasn't going to help us.

So-Called Medical Experts

Our mite infestation began in mid-Summer. As the weeks went on and we realized the problem was getting much worse, we began to trying things to fight the invasion. By the time we sought medical assistance, it was nearing the end of summer.

The constant bites had given us itchy, swollen bumps and rashes. We had also broken out in hives. A web site told us that certain medical drugs might be helpful against bird mites.

Right away, the doctor dismissed the idea that bird mites could be biting us. Without referring to us specifically, he explained that some people have "delusional bug syndrome" (experts call it "delusions of parasitosis"). Such people imagine they have parasites biting them, when there's nothing on them at all.

He then said matter-of-factly that bird mites never stay on humans for more than a few days, because they're only interested in birds. He finished by saying that he'd been taught this in medical school (BUT some research studies contradict this. See the appendix).

Still, he couldn't deny our very obvious skin problems, and the apparent bites we'd been experiencing. He did an exam, but didn't have a diagnosis yet.

What About Scabies?

Then the doctor discussed scabies. Scabies is the species of mite that commonly attack humans. But scabies mites are *very different* from bird mites. Scabies mites reproduce by burrowing *under* the skin to lay eggs, and the result, when the eggs hatch, is very intense *itching* (the word scabies is from the Latin "to scratch").
Unlike scabies, bird mites do NOT lay eggs under the skin.

They attach their eggs *to* the skin with protein glue. Or they attach the eggs to hairs (in the case of birds, to feathers). When the eggs hatch, the juveniles crawl around until they mature. Then the reproductive cycle starts again.

Bird mites get nourishment by biting the host. The largest part of a bird mite's tiny body is its jaws and biting mechanism. This is why such a very small creature can give such a painful bite.

Clearly, our symptoms did not match scabies. There was no intense itching.

The doctor decided to give us scabies medication anyway, just to see if it might help. He prescribed Permethrin. This pesticide cream is applied from head to toe, killing any scabies mites on the skin. A second application is made a few days later, to kill any new scabies mites that may have hatched under your skin.

Also at our request, he gave a prescription for oral Ivermectin (Stromectol). This drug is commonly used to kill internal parasites, such as roundworms. It supposedly will also kill scabies under your skin, by directly poisoning them.

We'd read about Ivermectin on the Internet. Some people said it had helped with their bird mite problem. (Sadly, a few online users seem addicted to the stuff, taking dose after dose without relief. That is risky. Excess use of this toxic drug can damage the liver).

In our case, after two rounds of treatment with each medication (Permethrin and Ivermectin), there was no improvement whatsoever. The biting and crawling was just as bad as ever. Clearly, scabies was not our problem. We were sure it was a bird mite problem, but the doctor still did not agree.

An Unknown Cause

On a return visit, the doc said the swollen bites and rashes were simply due to some unknown reaction, perhaps an allergy. He repeated what he had learned in medical school, 'bird mites don't stay on humans'.

Noticing the skin condition had become worse since the last visit, the doctor sent us to a dermatologist. That skin expert said the very same thing. Maybe it was an allergy, but it couldn't possibly be bird mites.

They said we were suffering from an "unknown cause", and the hives were described as *urticaria* (hives from an unknown cause). We were given some pills to reduce the rash and the hives. But it did nothing to reduce the mite bites and crawling. The medical experts had struck out!

Once again, we were on our own.

During those weeks of seeking a medical solution, we had decided to temporarily escape our home. By then, it was seriously overrun with bird mites. We got a room at a local hotel, one of those residential inn places.

Unfortunately, many mites came along for the ride (on clothing, in the car, and on us). So while at first things were marginally better, the hotel room soon got worse. The mites continued to multiply there. Also, the hotel did not launder the bedding every day for cost reasons. Sleep was increasingly difficult.

Clearly, we needed to learn more about fighting bird mites, and fast -- because things were quickly spiraling out of control.

Chapter Four: KNOW THE ENEMY

As we've mentioned, in the early weeks when we first began getting bites, we had no idea it was a bird mite problem. We just thought it was some minor annoyance, just random insect bites. We figured it was a temporary thing. Our slow response to the problem allowed the mites enough time to start reproducing, get a firm foothold, and spread themselves throughout our life. They soon fully established themselves, making us the center of their attention, as host of their parasite population.

In reading through research studies, we learned that when birds are present, bird mites are naturally attracted to them. That's why humans rarely encounter bird mites through normal outdoor activity. The mites' preferred targets (birds) are readily available throughout nature.

However, if no living creature other than humans is available (such as when mites are accidentally brought into a house, or a dead bird is next to a house, or an abandoned bird nest is by a house), then the hungry mites can enter the premises to seek out and adapt to human hosts. That's when they make themselves at home in YOUR home, and you become their preferred target.

Oh, It's Just Your Imagination

We also learned that it's possible for bird mites to go after *only one person* in a household, while the other family members seem immune and completely unaware of any problem. That can make things difficult for the solitary victim. That unlucky person not only has to deal with mites crawling and biting, but also the doubts of others. The others may assume the bird mite victim is just imagining things.

Why do bird mites sometimes single out certain people as hosts? It is believed that the *body chemistry* of one person can make them more attractive to the mites (this is well known to happen with mosquitoes, which will bite certain people more than others). In the case of mites, it's said that human females are more often victims of a mite problem. Again, this may be due to female body chemistry, or perhaps the diet of that person (if for example, they consume sugary sweets).

Relentless Invasion

In our case, the mites gradually infiltrated all our clothes and bedding.
We became their transport mechanism, spreading mites to all locations where we spent time (car, work, etc). We could feel them on us almost all the time, and especially at night. Their bites felt like random pinpricks, although sometimes a bite would be a hard jab, making us jump.

Despite our best efforts to clean our body from head to toe, along with cleaning clothing, home, and car -- there were always some mites and mite eggs that would survive. It's not easy to totally remove creatures that are microscopically small. Within a very short time, the population would rebound and activity would increase.

Mites are extremely sensitive to temperature changes and bodily chemical attractants. Scientists have found in experiments that they have a remarkable ability to quickly travel up to 100 yards to seek a victim. These diabolical creatures have built-in radar. They hone in on the heat and scent of their victims.

One very annoying behavior: mites can crawl up to the ceiling of a room. They wait there until they sense the victim's warmth or movement directly below, and then they drop down onto them. So, you might suddenly feel a mite land upon your scalp or neck as you walk through your home. (Later, we'll talk about a way to attack this.)

Research has shown that northern avian bird mites have developed near-total resistance to most pesticides (see research study #3 in the appendix). Resistance likely developed after many years of pesticide treatments on domestic chickens (mite-afflicted hens produce fewer eggs, so farmers liberally douse their broods with bug-killers. As a result, most bird mites now have pesticide immunity).

The creatures are incredibly tiny. Even against a bright white background, mites are barely visible, like the tiniest specks of black pepper. We actually saw several one day, during our infestation. We spotted them under bright light, on our clean white tile bathroom floor. When we tried to squash one tiny bug under a fingertip, it leapt instantly to another area on the floor. They have amazing survival skills.

More About Scabies vs. Bird Mites

In Chapter Three, we mentioned scabies mites. Let's now highlight the key differences between scabies mites and bird mites. While both creatures are mites, they have definite differences.

Scabies lay eggs *under* the skin, bites are small red spots, and extermination is relatively easy. On the other hand, avian (bird) mites lay eggs *on* the skin, bites may cause a large reaction (as they did with us), and extermination is usually difficult.

According to some reports, scabies mites are *more fragile* than bird mites. Hence it may be somewhat easier to eradicate them using common prescription treatments such as topical Pyrethrium cream (mild insecticide cream applied to entire body, left on skin for 12-14 hours, then washed off), or by taking an oral dose of an anti-parasite drug called Ivermectin (sold by Merck under the brand name Stromectol). The first dose is followed by a second dose, seven days later.

In the USA, the use of Ivermectin for scabies is considered "off label" by the FDA. In other words, it's not the suggested remedy, but is known to work on scabies.

Ivermectin ONLY works on Scabies mites, because it works *internally*. It zaps the scabies mites that have burrowed under the skin, and it kills the juveniles and females there.

Ivermectin is fairly toxic (that's why it kills internal scabies mites and certain other parasites). So it's best to take this medicine only as directed, and avoid excessive doses. But taken properly, it's a common anti-parasite drug used by humans worldwide. It's also given to dogs, horses and other animals to kill internal parasites.

So why doesn't Ivermectin kill bird mites? Again, bird mites live ON the skin, not UNDER skin or inside the body. Since they aren't inside you, they can't be hurt by a medicine which is inside your body.

Think you might have scabies? If you have already tried the two prescription drugs (Pyrethrium cream and/or Ivermectin-Stromectol) yet the scabies have not been eliminated, there are other possibilities to consider.

First, it is possible you *did* kill the scabies mites and eggs inside your body, but you got re-infected from clothes, bedding, home furnishings, etc. that were not fully disinfected. In this case, you need to more stringently clean, and then get re-treated by your doctor.

Second, it is possible that your scabies mites are resistant to the insecticide cream. In this case, follow the detailed solutions outlined in the chapters ahead for the elimination of bird mites, as this will also help to eliminate scabies mites.

Third, it is possible you got re-infected from a friend or family member. Scabies mites are spread by prolonged (or intimate) human contact. Avoid the infected party, while both of you get the treatment.

Know the Enemy

Before we list the ways to solve a bird mite problem in the following chapter, it's helpful to understand that bird mites go through several life stages. A bird mite starts out as an egg laid by a female.

Mites can reproduce in as little as 4 to 7 days, which is why their population can rise so quickly under ideal conditions. You do NOT want to provide those ideal conditions! But let's get back to our description of the life cycle. The egg is laid, and it soon hatches.

Juvenile bird mites do not bite. All they can do is crawl around at this stage (which can be very annoying). Once they reach maturity, the crawling mites become biting mites.

The moment a bird mite bites you, it gets all the nourishment it needs to reproduce. Now it just has to find a mite of the opposite sex, and soon more eggs will be laid. And the population keeps growing and growing.

Now that you know the facts, it's time to start fighting the problem.

Chapter Five: ATTACK THE MITES

Let's begin with a one sentence summary of what must happen.

Kill all the bird mites and mite eggs you can, while making it as difficult as possible for any survivors to remain in your environment.

Here are the three basic steps to eradicate a population of bird mites. As we discovered, some of these methods work better than others, but when combined, they are far more effective.

1. Repel them (adjust environment & use mite irritants)
2. Escape them (plastic barriers, door seals, etc.)
3. Destroy them (specific substances and practices)

Now let's explore these effective mite-fighting strategies in detail.

Solving the Bird Mite Problem

There is no single "magic bullet" on the list above that will solve a bird mite infestation. This is because the creatures are so resourceful. We personally tried dozens of things to get rid of the mites. Now we share the exact combination that worked so well for us.

- Indoor environmental changes
- Indoor treatments
- Body modifications
- Cleaning routines
- Habitat modifications

Keep in mind, this is an all-out war.

As a warrior, you do whatever it takes to win the war. Half-hearted measures may win a battle, but they won't get you total victory. To become completely mite-free, you need to take action and do what it takes to win.

Scientists say the life span of bird mites (when no host is available) is 90 days. However, some reports say mites can survive for up to six months, on stored clothing and household items. We agree with the longer estimate. Some mites survived on clothing inside plastic storage bags in our home for more than 90 days, which caused us to have a brief, minor re-infestation.
To be completely safe, conservatively figure the life span of bird mites with no host available to be *six months.*

No More Fibers

Keeping that six month lifespan in mind, we went to work on our bird mite problem. We know that in nature, mites live, feed and reproduce on birds. Birds are covered with natural fibers (feathers). Bird mites have evolved to grasp the shafts of these fibers and hold on, despite burning hot sunshine, drenching rains, and fierce winds. In fact, microscopic photos show them doing just that. Female avian mites attach their eggs to these fiber shafts (or the bird skin) with protein glue. The eggs soon hatch, continuing the infestation.

Now look around your home. You probably have carpeting, fabric furniture, and maybe some throw pillows or a blanket on the couch.

Your bedding and pillow are made of fabric. Your mattress and box springs are fabric-covered. You might have fabric window treatments. All this fabric material is loaded with fibers, which is to bird mites like home sweet home.

What can you do? Well before we answer that question, here's a crazy story to consider.

A Squirrely Situation

Let's imagine you own some land. It contains a small forest. Your little forest has a big problem: it's infested with rabid, biting squirrels. You want to get rid of all those nasty biting squirrels, but they're too small and too quick to catch, shoot, or trap. And they're completely resistant to poisons.

So what do you do? Well, here's a radical idea -- you get rid of the trees!
You hire a lumberjack to chop down all the trees, leaving nothing but bare ground. So what happens to those

nasty squirrels? They're gone. This is because it is the squirrel's nature to live in and around trees. Trees are where squirrels nest, reproduce, and hibernate. They do not like the bare ground and they won't live on bare ground. They will go elsewhere in search of trees, or else they will slowly die off.

Yes, it's radical to chop down all the trees (tree huggers won't like that), but it does solve the squirrel problem. And once the squirrels are all gone, you can always plant more trees and get your forest back again.

So what does this story have to do with bird mites?

Remember, their natural habitat is among fibers. That's where they prefer to live and reproduce, clinging to microscopic fiber shafts. Get rid of the fibers, and you have made the environment much, much less attractive to mites.

Store or Remove the Fabric

By temporarily removing (or sealing up) ALL the fabric (especially any natural fibers, such as cotton or wool) in your living and sleeping areas, you make it far more difficult for bird mites to remain there.

Once we chose this plan of action (explained in the pages ahead), we bit the bullet and checked out of the hotel, to return to our heavily infested home. We knew we'd suffer from some immediate bites, but we were determined to start fixing the problem. First, we stopped by the home improvement store and then the local Wal-Mart, and bought some items.

Here is Shopping List #1. There are five more Shopping Lists ahead in the book. Eventually, you may wish to buy all suggested products to apply all the strategies we recommend. Note: if the word "optional" appears by an item, you may not need it, unless you wish to try every option.

Shopping List #1
(for the average-sized home)

- One dozen large, clear plastic dropcloths (9 x 12 feet is a good size)
- Several rolls of clear packing tape
- One carton of Carpet Protection Film, if you have wall-to-wall carpeting (buy this at Home Depot or Amazon.com)
- A box of large black plastic trash bags
- Five boxes of white plastic kitchen trash bags (you may need more or less)
- Several dozen replacement bags for your vacuum cleaner
- Polyester bedding, pillow, and bath towels (all or mostly polyester, with little or no cotton)
- Six empty plastic spray bottles
- Six bottles of 85%-95% strength isopropyl rubbing alcohol (NOT 60%-70%)

In the next chapter, we'll explain how to modify your living spaces to help eliminate mites.

Chapter Six: CLEAN AND SEAL UP

Our home had mostly hardwood floors, covered with area rugs.

We began the process of fabric removal by rolling up the rugs. Then we wrapped the rolled-up rugs in plastic drop cloths, taping the seams to tightly seal the rugs inside. We then stored these sealed-up rugs in our basement and garage (they can also be stored, rolled up, in the same room they came from, if space is limited).

Next, the couch and chair were looking old anyway. So we put those out with the trash (please do not donate infested furniture to Goodwill). We replaced the couch and chair with affordable leather furniture (bird mites do not like leather – it's like bare skin to them).

Can't afford new furniture? Then seal your fabric furniture in plastic film -- as we describe later in this chapter.

A Few Words about Floors

Hard, non-carpeted floors are best to discourage mite activity. The very best floor is *tile or stone*, as it offers mites very few places to hide. Tile and stone are also very easy to clean. Linoleum is quite good, depending on how many seams it has (seams are where mites hide). The third best surface is hardwood, as lots of mites can hide in its crevices. The worst type of floor to have is carpeting, as the fabric quickly becomes infested with mites and eggs. Carpet is also the toughest to keep clean.

Whatever you do, please *do not* use a wet cleaning machine on your carpet to remove mites! The hot water won't kill any bird mites, but it will cause the population to explode and the mite activity will rapidly increase. *Moisture and humidity should be strictly avoided -- this energizes bird mites.*

Likewise, avoid using water or wet mops to clean hard floors. Vacuuming and dry mopping (Swiffer) are far better. One exception: you may occasionally mop a tile floor, or clean a bathroom counter, using a strong bleach + hot water solution.

Wall-to-Wall Carpet

Here's how to deal with a room that has tacked-down wall-to-wall carpet. One of our rooms had wall-to-wall. Rather than pull it up or remove it, we sealed it in place. This is why the shopping list includes a roll of adhesive Carpet Protection Film (sold at Home Depot and Amazon.com) The roll of two-foot wide, clear plastic film is sticky on one side. You unroll the stuff sticky side down. It adheres to the carpet very effectively and seals it completely. It's commonly used by housepainters and construction workers to protect carpeting.
Be sure to read the instructions, as there's a trick to getting it to unroll smoothly and lay flat on the carpet.

It's easier if two people do it. But you can manage it fine by yourself, with a little practice. You'll need scissors or a knife to cut the film, of course.

Since the film is two feet wide, you need to lay down five (or six) passes in order to completely seal up the average-size room carpet. Overlap each strip slightly with the next, to completely seal the rug. You'll also need to seal the rug's edges against the baseboards on all four walls (clear plastic packing tape can be used to do this). If you mess up, and leave a gap or opening somewhere on the rug, no worries. Just apply a piece of clear tape, or another layer of carpet film, to seal it completely. Since it's clear, nobody will notice an extra layer or two.

Presto, the carpet on the floor is sealed tight under clear plastic. Any mites and mite eggs in the rug will remain trapped in there, and will all be dead in six months (although we left our carpet film in place for a full year). And we guarantee you, if your home has a bird mite problem, there are mites and eggs hiding in your carpet. The good news – after six months, they'll be deceased and completely harmless.

The makers of the carpet film recommend it be removed from a rug in 30 days. We kept the film on our carpet for a full year, and never had any problem. Our wall-to-wall carpet was perfectly fine when we finally peeled off the stuff, with no residue or damage. In fact, the rug looked beautiful. (Of course, we can't make promises about your rugs, nor can we be held liable for damages. Some rugs may be more delicate than ours.)

What to Tell Others

At this point, you may be freaking out. "What do I tell my friends who visit my home (or my landlord) about the plastic film on the carpet?!"

Well, our story was this: "Allergies are a real problem. This plastic really helps to deal with it, and it's perfectly safe for the carpet."

Of course, we never said that WE had any allergy! But that story seemed to settle the issue for everyone. (Had we wanted to be totally upfront, we could have said the plastic was to stop mites -- and most people would assume we meant *dust mites*. Those are widely known to live in carpets.)

As far as keeping the surface of the carpet film clean, the vacuum cleaner didn't work – it got stuck on the plastic surface. So we used a dry Swiffer dust mop (NOT a wet mop) to pick up any dust and dirt. This worked well.

Next, the Bedroom

Our bedroom was another matter entirely. The mattress and box spring were fully infested with bird mites, as was the area rug on the floor. Now it was time to deal with the problem. That room was ground zero with the bird mite problem, and it was no good fixing the rest of the place if we didn't deal with the worst room.

So off we went to the local mattress store and ordered a new set. We made sure the price included delivery AND takeaway of the old set, and a new bed frame.

When the truck arrived, we had the men set up the new bed in our downstairs family room (the room with the already sealed carpet film). Then we took the men upstairs to haul away the old bed set.

If anyone might still be thinking our bird mite problem was one big hallucination or delusion – or an overactive imagination – what happened next is something we will never forget. It proved to us that our problem was frighteningly real.

As we watched the men reach down to pick up our old bed, they both flinched dramatically, jumped and both said "Ouch! OW!" Of course, we instantly felt awful, realizing they were getting bitten by mites! Believe it or not, we hadn't considered that, since we felt the mites were our personal enemy and would only attack us. After all, the pest control guy who visited our home hadn't gotten a single bite. But this room was the hot zone for the mite problem and we should have known better. Stupid, we know. Especially stupid, in retrospect.

We would guess anyone whose job it is to remove old beds must see a few unpleasant things from time to time. In our case, the bed still looked brand new. But the bird mites infesting it were virtually invisible of course.

These delivery men were pretty tough dudes. After the initial bites, one shrugged and said, "That has to be static shocks. It's pretty dry in here." The other one said "I'm not so sure about that" and gave us a look. "If those are static shocks, they're the worst I've ever felt".

As they hustled the bed down the stairs, we saw them both flinch hard, several more times. They went out the door and tossed the bed into the back of their pickup truck. We gave them a very healthy tip.

We still feel bad about that situation. But if there's anything positive to say about it, it removed any shred of doubt that there was a very real, very obnoxious bird mite infestation.

With the old bed gone, we reluctantly went back into the bedroom. We first rolled up the area rug (and got many more hard, nasty bites in the process). We sealed that infested rug tightly inside a plastic dropcloth, making sure to close up all the seams carefully with tape, and set the rolled-up rug against one wall.

Clean Out the Closets

With the infested bed and rug taken care of, we thoroughly vacuumed every square inch of the floor. Then we immediately removed the vacuum cleaner bag, double bagging it in white plastic trash bags, and tossed it into a garbage can outside.

Now the room was more bearable, although we were still getting an occasional bite. We now turned to the closets, which were stuffed with clothes. This is where the large plastic trash bags came into play.

We took all the clothes out of the closets and dressers, stuffing it all in large black plastic bags, and sealed those tightly. If there was any doubt, we double-bagged the items. Lastly, we did the same with all the towels and bedding in the master bath and linen closet.

We would not enter that bedroom or bathroom again for six months, until we knew that all mites and eggs in the sealed up rug, clothing, and linens were completely dead and harmless.

Lastly, we closed the door to the bedroom, and using clear plastic tape, sealed all four edges of the door around the door frame. Now it would just take time for that "hot zone" to become stone cold. Things were progressing!

What to Wear

You may be wondering what we did about our clothes, towels and bedding. Well, remember what we said about bird mites preferring NATURAL fibers like cotton and wool. Most everything we bagged up for storage was either cotton or wool, which we like to wear as they are comfortable fabrics. Unfortunately, bird mites love it too.

We took another trip to the local Wal-Mart. There we purchased a supply of polyester clothing, socks, underwear, and so on. We even bought their cheap polyester athletic shoes, and a nylon outerwear jacket. If you're a fashion king or queen, you may be cringing. Don't dismiss polyester clothing. Go to the store and see what it looks like. Most of what we bought not only looked good, but we even got compliments on some of the items.

Shopping List #2

- Polyester and/or nylon clothing
- Polyester undergarments
- Polyester socks
- Polyester blend bed sheets/pillow cases (two sets)
- Polyester blanket
- Inexpensive athletic shoes (polyester)
- Nylon outerwear jackets
- Polyester bath towels and washcloths
- Polyester dish towels for the kitchen

We can say from direct experience that mites are far less interested in infesting the man-made fabrics such as polyester, rayon, and nylon (just as squirrels don't like to live in plastic trees).

As we said, we prefer to wear natural cotton clothing. But it was a no-brainer to store those away and switch to polyester, if it helped solve our mite problem. And yes, it did help.

By the way, many other items at Wal-Mart can be a big help in a bird mite battle. More about that later. (We don't own stock in Wal-Mart or have a connection with them, other than as a shopper. Many items can be found at other stores such as Target.)

Wrapping a Bed in Plastic

Until the mites were gone from our bedroom, we would be sleeping on the new bed in the family room, simply because the bedroom was so badly infested. You may not need to temporarily change the room you sleep in, if your infestation isn't as severe as ours. But you still need to do the following bed treatment.

The new bed needed to be made mite-resistant, and this is something you must do, regardless of the room you sleep in. Again, grab the trusty roll of carpet protection film, but this time you'll use it to seal up the mattress and then the box spring (separately), so they are each completely encased in plastic film.

Begin by completely covering one face of the mattress with the adhesive film. Then flip the mattress over and cover the other side of the mattress with the carpet protection film. Next, set the mattress on one edge and apply plastic film to the three exposed sides (top, bottom, and side) of the mattress, making sure to overlap the film onto the faces of the mattress, for a complete seal. Finally, turn it onto the other edge, and finish sealing the last side.

Now repeat the entire same process with the box spring, sealing it in plastic -- top, bottom, sides and ends.

Once you've done this, put the box spring in the bed frame, and place the mattress on top of it.

(If you're working by yourself, this process is easiest if your bed is a smaller model, such as a twin set. If you have a queen size or larger bed, you may need some help for this process.)

By the way, if you have fabric couches or chairs you must keep, use the same procedure to wrap the furniture all over in carpet protection film, or else use plastic dropcloths and clear tape on them -- top, bottom and sides.

Even if you put the items in storage somewhere for six months, it's best to seal them in plastic first, to avoid spreading mites to other storage units.

Bagging Up Pillows

The next step is to double-bag your bare pillow(s) in white plastic trash bags. After double-bagging them, slip a polyester pillowcase over the plastic bag.

Mites love to hide within pillows, especially those containing natural fibers. Having a pillow that's encased in plastic solves this problem. We suggest using two cloth pillowcases on each pillow, as this will makes sleeping more comfortable. The plastic bag inside will make a slight crinkling noise when you rest your head on the pillow, but we got used to it quickly.

Your pillowcases, fitted sheet, top sheet and blanket(s) should all be made of polyester fabric (at least an 80-20 polyester-cotton blend). Buy at least two complete sets of bedding, so one set can be laundered while the other set is being used.

There was a special bedtime routine we carefully followed every night to help keep the bed mite-free, and we'll explain that later.

Clutter and Paper

One more thing about home furnishings. Mites love paper and they love clutter. All those nooks and crannies in piles of paper and household clutter are great places for mites to hang out. So any stacks of paper, magazines, bills, receipts, etc. must also be bagged in plastic and stored away. No more clutter anywhere!

All the furnishings must be sealed up and put away too. All closets must be emptied, and the contents stored in tightly sealed plastic bags (double bagging is highly recommended). You want bare floors and bare surfaces everywhere, as much as possible.

If your house is stacked high with stuff and you lack storage space, consider renting a storage unit. But please don't allow bird mites to infest other people's storage units. Seal up everything in plastic, before you put it in storage. Plan to leave it there, untouched and unopened, for at least six months. Then all the mites and eggs within it will be completely dead.

Chairs

Obviously you need a chair (or several) to sit on to eat your meals, read this book, watch TV, surf the web, play video games, and so on. Fabric chairs tend to harbor mites like crazy. Sit on one in an infested home, and soon you'll feel the mites crawling around your pelvic area, and then all over you.

The solution we found was to store away the fabric chairs and buy a few metal folding chairs. They're affordable at Target or Wal-Mart. Metal is unfriendly to mites, although even a metal chair has seams and crevices where mites can hide.

Each day before using a metal chair, give it a thorough spray down with isopropyl alcohol, using one of the spray bottles you bought.

90%+ strength rubbing alcohol is one of the few products we found that consistently repelled bird mites. However, weaker alcohol solutions (60-70%) are NO GOOD because of their high water content. Mites thrive on water. So avoid the low-strength rubbing alcohol and never use water-based cleaners, such as Windex or Formula 409.

Here is how to prepare the chair. Each time before sitting on a metal chair, spray a mist of alcohol on the front, back, sides, legs and (flip it over) *under* the seat. Alcohol evaporates fast, leaving you with a clean, mite-free chair. What a pleasure!

Plastic Spray Bottles

Speaking of spray bottles and high-strength isopropyl alcohol, we suggest you keep five or six spray bottles filled at all times.

Keep one by your bed, another by your favorite chair, another in the kitchen, one in the bathroom, perhaps one at your workplace, and anywhere else you spend time. Keep a bottle within arm's reach, so you can blast it at mites wherever you notice them.

Already, you're making lifestyle changes that are very helpful to permanently eradicate bird mites from your home. There's more to come.

Chapter Seven: SET YOUR ROUTINES

If you've been paying attention, you've noticed that we have mentioned water as a negative factor, one you should avoid. Humidity of any kind is like rocket fuel for mites, because it makes them far more active. So you must limit the moisture and humidity in your home, as much as possible.

Unfortunately for us, our infestation was at its worst in late summer and early fall. There also was massive amounts of rainfall during that time. The air became very humid, yet it was also quite cool. So we were unable to run our air conditioning to reduce indoor humidity. Cool, humid weather is ideal for the mites. In our case, they began to reproduce like crazy.

Our ignorance about mite behavior made things even worse. We assumed that if we really washed the floors, that would help get rid of the bugs. So we scrubbed every floor surface with a wet mop. This was the one of the worst things we could have done. It helped the bird mite population to massively grow in no time.

The best thing is to keep your floors completely water-free! And keep the indoor humidity as low as possible, at all times. In northern climates, it is often very dry in the winter. In our case, at the coldest times of winter we noticed a substantial reduction in mite activity. This was because our indoor air became bone dry.

Sources of Indoor Humidity

You can't control the weather outside. In our area (northern US), three seasons can have high humidity: Spring, Summer, and Fall. Summer is actually not so bad, because we can run the air conditioning, which lowers the humidity. But Spring and Fall were challenging times due to damp weather.

If you live in a mostly dry region such as the Southwest US, that's a big plus. But if you're located in a humid region, such as the Southeast US, consider buying a few dehumidifiers. Place them in different areas of your home.

An electric dishwasher or top-loading clothes washer will add lots of humidity to the air. Steamy, moist air pours out of these units when they run -- and especially at the end of the cycle, when you open the unit. Luckily, our kitchen had a powerful exhaust fan, which we'd run while using the dishwasher.

Here's a tip about the dishwasher. Following the rinse cycle, most dishwashers cycle to "dry" mode. In this mode, an internal fan pushes the steamy air out into the room, helping to dry the dishes inside the machine. We would always make sure to manually shut off the machine, at the end of the rinse cycle. We did this by manually advancing the control knob to "off", preventing it from going to "dry" mode. That way, steamy air stays inside the unit, where it condenses.

After about an hour, when the door is cool to the touch, that's when to unload the dishes. This helps keep humidity low in the home.

In the case of the clothes washer, we noticed a huge improvement when we finally got rid of our top-loading machine and bought a modern front-loader. A front-loading machine is actually a major key in ridding your life of bird mites. We cover this in detail ahead.

Bathroom Humidity

Showers and baths generate humid air, too. If you have a bathroom exhaust fan, by all means use it. If your bathroom does not have an exhaust fan, consider having one installed. It will make a big difference.

Also, keep the bathroom door closed as much as possible, to keep the humid air from getting into the rest of your home. After your bath or shower is done and you exit the bathroom, close the door behind you.

Cleaning Your Home

Since moisture and humid air encourage bird mite activity in your home, how do you clean floors and other surfaces? And by the way, it is vital that you clean your home regularly.

Some "experts" suggest mopping the floors every single day to fight mites. If you've been following our advice so far, you know this is a bad idea.

On the other hand, we do encourage *very frequent vacuuming* of every room in your home, every few days. Each time before you vacuum, put a new bag in the machine. Afterwards, immediately remove it from the machine, double-bag in plastic trash bags, and toss the bag in an outside trash can.

If it's not possible to vacuum certain rooms (for example, if a room has wall-to-wall covered with plastic film), then use a DRY Swiffer dust mop with a disposable pad (never a wet pad). As soon as you are done, double-bag the dry pad and dispose of it in an outside can.

Vacuuming daily helps remove bird mite eggs, juvenile mites, and some of the mature mites on your floors. It also removes dust, hair, and debris you can't see -- which mites find very inviting.

Cleaning the Bathrooms

One helpful trick after your bath or shower is to spray down the shower or
tub area with a heavy mist of straight ammonia. *Caution! Ammonia is strong stuff, so avoid inhaling the fumes.*

To do this, fill a new spray bottle with straight ammonia, and leave it in your bathroom. *Be sure to clearly label the bottle, perhaps with a red marker, so you know it's ammonia!*

After every shower or bath (and after you've dried off and are ready to exit the bathroom), grab the bottle and douse the shower stall or tub area with liberal sprays of the ammonia.

It is best if you close the shower door (or curtains) FIRST. Then, reach up and aim the sprayer over the top. In this way, the mist will drift down in the enclosed space. This way, you won't be engulfed in ammonia fumes but the shower or tub area gets a concentrated blast. The fumes will dissipate in a while, having killed some mites in the area. Added benefit: over time, the daily ammonia spray will totally eliminate all traces of mold and mildew in your shower or tub area, leaving it sparkling clean.

<u>Caution</u>: *never mix bleach and ammonia together, or use them both at the same time. The combination will cause hazardous fumes.*

You should also vacuum the bathroom floor when you vacuum the rest of the house.

Here's an extra step to try after shower or bath. Just before exiting the bathroom, mist the tile floor with high strength isopropyl alcohol from your alcohol spray bottle. Also mist the toilet, including the open and closed seat, to zap any mites that may be hiding there.

Returning Home

During the long months when our home, car, and workplace were infested with bird mites, we had a regular routine upon arriving home at night. After eight or ten hours away from home, we'd feel mites crawling on us. So we kept a supply of plastic trash bags right inside the front door. Upon stepping inside the door, we'd immediately disrobe and put every stitch of clothing in plastic bags, which we'd close tightly. Those clothes would be washed later.

Shoes went in a separate bag, to be washed or sprayed with alcohol later, before wearing them again. More about shoes in a moment.

After bagging the clothes and shoes, a quick shower would follow. Then we'd put on clean clothes for the evening. This made life a little more pleasant. It significantly reduced the mites on us, at least for a little while.

Dealing with Shoes

Here's an important rule: never walk around at home with bare feet. The warmth of your feet on the floor acts like a magnet for mites. Always wear something on your feet such as sandals, even if you get out of bed at night for a glass of water. Wear flip-flops or sandals when you head to and from the shower. Slip them off just before you step into the shower, and as soon as you step out, put them back on.

Bird mites are drawn to shoes, which is very annoying. We often felt them crawling around in there and sometimes biting us there too.

Unfortunately, it's not easy to toss most footwear in a washing machine (although we did this with athletic shoes, sometimes). For a while we were buying pairs of cheap athletic shoes at Wal-Mart, and bagging them for periods of time when they'd get infested. But that was a costly solution.

The cheap shoes survived the wash OK, but drying them took forever. And often, live mites would remain in the shoes even after washing them, since the shoes have so many crevices where they can hide.

The Shoe Solution

Here's how we finally solved the shoe dilemma. We only wore shoes that have easily *removable insoles* (the insole is the inner part of the shoe, the part your foot rests on). One brand with removable insoles is New Balance. That company makes leather as well as athletic shoes with removable insoles (not glued down). Also, some of the Nike athletic shoes have removable insoles.

Here's why this matters: mites usually hide under and around the insole. If you can't remove the insole, you'll never zap all the mites inside the shoe before wearing it the next time.

This is the shoe cleaning routine we suggest you follow.

Each morning, before putting on a pair of shoes, get rid of any lint that's inside. To do this, remove the insoles one at a time. Using your hand, brush off each insole over a wastebasket to remove any bits of lint or fuzz on the insole (which attract mites). Pay special attention to the edges of the insole, removing every bit of lint.

Once the insole is clean, take a spray bottle of high strength alcohol and soak the top and the bottom of the insole. Set it aside. Next, spray the shoe. First, spray the outside -- top, sides, and bottom of the shoe. Then spray the inside of the shoe (don't put the insole back in yet). Set everything aside to dry, in a clean spot (such as on a table) until the alcohol fully evaporates, which only takes a few minutes. And don't worry about putting shoes on the table -- the alcohol spray has sterilized them.

Once the shoes and insoles are dry, there's a trick to put on the shoes without getting mites inside. First, slip off one of your sandals or flip flops (you ARE wearing those and not going barefoot, right?) Then slip on a clean sock, keeping your foot off the floor. Insert an insole into one shoe, and then slip that shoe on your foot. Follow the same process for the other foot. This brief routine keeps your bare feet off the floor, and gives you mite-free footwear to start the day. After a bit of practice it only takes a few minutes.

During the day, you may feel mites crawling inside one or both shoes, or even feel a bite or two. The bugs seem to gravitate there, perhaps because of warmth and natural moisture. If you feel mites, here's a quick fix. Take off the shoe and give it another good spraying inside with alcohol, and spray your sock (still on your foot) lightly, as well. Keep your foot off the floor while you let the sock and shoe dry, which happens quickly. Then slip the shoe back on. This usually stops any mite activity. An added benefit to spraying your shoes like this – your feet will always smell fresh!

If you notice mites jumping on your feet or legs while you are in a certain area of your home, mist some alcohol on the floor area that surrounds you, in a 360 degree pattern.

Chapter Eight: DO THE LAUNDRY

If you have a serious bird mite infestation, you may want to do laundry on a frequent basis -- possibly, every single day.

One of the most important things we did in retrospect was to junk our old top-loading washer and buy a modern front-loader with a *steam cycle*. What an amazing difference this made!

The brand we chose was Samsung, but other companies make similar models. Just be sure it has a *steam cleaning cycle*. (You can also get a dryer with steam, which we bought later. But a dryer with steam isn't essential. Our regular old dryer worked fine, for quite a while.)

The new washer used far less water, and put only a minimal amount of humidity into the air, compared to our old machine. And our old washer discharged many gallons of steaming water every time it did a load. That hot water would slowly drain into the laundry sink, putting more moisture into the air, fueling mite activity. The new washer's water output was minimal. It went down the drain fast and didn't affect the indoor humidity.

Most importantly, the new machine did a far better job of cleaning clothes and bedding. With the old washer, a significant number of mites always seemed to survive the wash and dry cycle. Not many survived going through the new washer, and soon (thanks also to the other steps outlined in the book) there were no mites at all in our clothes or bedding!

Initially, before we got the steam washer, we used a few mite-zapping laundry additives that we'd read about online. They did help kill some mites for a while, but the bugs always seemed to adapt and bounce back. We'd put on supposedly clean, freshly washed items, and immediately feel mites. Arrgh! Or we'd climb into bed on freshly washed sheets, and right away, mites would start crawling on us. Very, very frustrating.

For the record, we'll share some laundry additives we tried, although we made them "optional" on the shopping list here. You are welcome to try them, if you wish.

Shopping List #3

- One or more gallons of laundry bleach
- Three to five quarts of ammonia (plain or lemon scent)
- Several boxes of Borax powder (NOT boric acid) Borax boosts detergent (and kills mites). It's in the detergent aisle at Wal-Mart.
- A few more empty spray bottles to fill with ammonia (label the bottles, and never mix bleach with ammonia)

- XTreme Cleen or another powerful cleaning additive (optional)
- Benzyl benzoate (optional)

Laundry Additives

The first laundry additive we tried was in our old top-loading machine. This product cannot be used in a front-loader, since it must be diluted in plenty of water. Front loaders don't use much water. The product was called XTreme Kleen.

To use this product, you first put clothes in the machine and let the washer tub fill up with hot water. Then, you stop the cycle and open the lid. Pour in a *diluted* amount of XTreme Cleen (never use full-strength, as it may damage clothes. And use care handling it -- direct contact can burn the skin). Keep it well out of the reach of children, too.

Once you've added the diluted XTreme Kleen product to the washer, pause the machine and let the load soak in the hot water for about an hour. This will kill off mites in the clothes. Then, restart the machine and let it run on through.

Did this product work? Yes, it seemed to help for a while. But all that steaming hot water put humidity into the air, which wasn't helpful. And an increasing number of mites seemed to survive, as time went by (they have amazing adaptability to many chemical products).

After about two months of using this product, the top-loader developed a serious leak inside somewhere. Perhaps the powerful product melted one of the internal parts? Or maybe the machine just broke down. We do not know. In any case, we stopped using the product. And we ordered the new front-loading washer.

You may not choose to use Xtreme Cleen. There are other high-powered cleaning liquids on the market, some touting an "natural organic formula". None of those other product had much effect, in our experience.

Benzyl Benzoate

Another laundry additive we used for a number of months was benzyl benzoate. It is neither a cleaning agent nor a disinfectant. It's a mite repellent.

To use this product, add a small amount of benzyl benzoate to the wash during the final rinse cycle. It is clear and odorless, and seems to do nothing. But when you put the clothes in the dryer, heat activates the stuff. It creates strong fumes in the dryer to kill or repel mites in your clothes. The pine-tar scent of heat-activated benzyl benzoate is unusual. A slight odor may remain on your clothes after drying (personally, we didn't mind it). Also, should you open the dryer door before the clothes are fully dry, you may see some white smoke drift out.

No worries, that's the active benzyl benzoate doing its thing. Once the clothes are fully dry, there's no more smoke.

Interestingly, before medical science discovered drugs like Permethrin to combat scabies, the old-time remedy was to apply a diluted solution of benzyl benzoate to the body. Unfortunately, that does not work with bird mites (nor was it very effective for scabies either). And it may cause side effects when used on the skin.

Suggested Daily Laundry Routine

As we've stated, a front-loading washer with a steam cycle is extremely helpful for mite reduction.

If you get a steam machine, be sure to wash clothes and bedding using the highest wash settings:

- Sanitize
- Steam
- "Activ Fresh" (adds silver ions to disinfect)
- Extra Hot water
- High Spin
- Heavy Soil Level.

These are all the Samsung washer settings we used. Your machine settings may be different. Just use the highest wash settings available. This will kill lots of mites and get your clothes really clean.

The full Samsung wash cycle described above takes over two hours per load. But unlike the old machine, which we'd have to babysit, pour in additives, stop the unit, start it again, etc. -- now we could just let it run.

Never overfill the washer. Cleaning is most effective when the machine isn't overloaded. You want the steam to reach all the clothes. If the machine is packed full, the steam can't penetrate everything, so some mites will survive. Give your washer some room, and it will kill more mites for you.

Along with detergent, we always added the following products:

FOR WHITES (bedding and towels), always use bleach.

FOR DARK LOADS, skip the bleach. Instead, use one-half cup ammonia (just pour it on the clothes -- don't use the dispenser). NEVER MIX bleach and ammonia -- it creates harmful fumes.

FOR ALL LOADS, add half-cup Borax powder (NOT boric acid). Borax kills bird mites. Find it in the detergent aisle at Wal-Mart.

Be sure to completely dry all your clothes and bedding, using the high heat setting on your dryer. This also helps kill mites.

Optional Idea for the Dryer

Before we got the new *steam dryer* (which blasts clothes with sterilizing steam as they dry), we sometimes tried a special treatment using the old dryer to zap any mites hiding in there. (Yes, some mites will survive the heat inside a clothes dryer.)

NOTE: we only offer this tip as optional info. USE CAUTION, it might void your warranty and damage your dryer.

Before putting in a load to dry, we'd run the dryer empty for a full minute or two, to get it nice and hot inside. Then, we'd grab a spray bottle of straight ammonia, open the dryer door, and shoot a few blasts inside, and quickly slam the door shut. The dryer heat would instantly vaporize the ammonia. Those powerful fumes would kill hidden mites in the machine. We'd let it cook for a minute or two. Then we'd turn on the dryer for a minute, to send the ammonia fumes to the exhaust vent outdoors. Lastly, we'd open the door, toss in the wet laundry load, and run the dryer as usual.

AGAIN we mention, this ammonia treatment could damage your dryer. We didn't care about our dryer much, as we were planning to get a new dryer. But it did seem to help eradicate the mites that somehow survived in our clothes after washing and drying them.

One more laundry suggestion: when your clothes and bedding are completely dry, remove them from the dryer, immediately fold them and insert them into plastic trash bags. Seal them until ready to wear. This helps keep clean laundry items mite-free.

If your budget is limited and a new washer with a steam cycle is out of the question, here's an alternate idea. After washing and drying your clothes, iron them with a steam iron that's set to high heat. This will also help kill mites remaining in the fabric.

Chapter Nine: GET TO BED

As you've noticed, we recommend a non-stop, multi-step effort to fully eliminate bird mites.

This means you can't skip a day or slack off, just because you're feeling a little tired. Don't expect the mites to do the same. This infernal pest has survived for millennia because it has the ability to quickly adapt to conditions that would kill off lesser bugs. And bird mites are relentless in seeking you, as their host. You are their food source and the place for them to lay eggs and reproduce. To halt their progress and eventually kill them off, you must make a daily effort and not skip steps or blow off the regular routine.

The resources we are sharing are definitely not "the lazy man's way" to get rid of mites. Frankly, there is no such thing. Getting rid of bird mites takes hard work, dedication, some guts, and determination to win. But the steps DO WORK. Stay with them and you will get results.

When Going to Bed Each Night

It's human nature that we take for granted the small blessings in life, until they are taken away. One such small blessing that countless millions of people expect is a peaceful night of rest, without interruption or turmoil.

But for anyone suffering with a bird mite infestation, a good night's sleep can suddenly become a rare and precious commodity.

We remember early in the bird mite attack, how amazed and lucky we'd feel when waking up on those rare mornings, having slept the whole night through without mites torturing us. Those nights were very few and far between. Most of the time, sleep time was hellish, with highly active, crawling and biting mites all over us until dawn.

There were nights we'd wearily climb out of bed at 3AM to change all of the bedding, or vacuum the bed, hoping to reduce that night's onslaught. Over time, we developed a set routine that prepared the bed for a reasonably good night of sleep, by reducing the mite annoyance. Now we share that effective routine with you.

First, we assume you already covered your mattress and box spring set with carpet protection film, as outlined in Chapter Six. Also, your pillow(s) should be bagged in plastic. You'll need a freshly laundered set of polyester-blend bedding (NOT all-cotton) stored in a sealed, clean, plastic trash bag, and ready to use.

To repeat, it's important to use sheets, blanket and pillowcases that are 100% polyester or a blend of 80-20 poly-cotton. This discourages mite activity. They dislike man-made fibers.

Prep your bed early each evening, a few hours before bedtime. Mites harbor during the daylight hours in cracks, crevices and tight spaces. Then at night, they emerge and get much more active, crawling and biting. Beds unfortunately contain many hiding places for mites: under the mattress, under the box spring, and in the bed frame. So each evening, your first step is to zap all the mites that may be hiding in your bed.

This process is pretty easy to do yourself if you have a small bed, such as a twin or full set. But if you have a queen or king, you will definitely need help with this. But don't neglect to do this every night -- it makes a big difference! Here's what to do.

How to Zap the Bed Before Bedtime

The bed should be bare at this point. Just the plastic-covered mattress, box spring, and the bed frame. Set the pillow(s) on a nearby chair or table (not on the floor).

Grab two spray bottles containing high-strength isopropyl alcohol. Hold one in each hand (imagine you're a gunslinger in the old West).

Slowly walk around the bed, completely misting all four sides and the top of the mattress. No need to drench the plastic film, just lightly mist it all over. Let it sit for five minutes until dry.

Next, lift the mattress off the bed, and stand it up on one end, so it rests on the floor by the bed. Now spray the underside of the mattress. Next, spray the top of the box spring, which is still in the bed frame. No need to wait for that to dry.

Now lift the box spring out of the bed frame, and stand it up on one end on the floor, next to the mattress (lean it again a wall if necessary). Mist the underside of the box spring with alcohol.

And now, walk around the bed frame, carefully misting every corner and part of it. Then lift up one end of the bed frame, and stand it up so the underside is facing you (lean it against a wall). Spray the underside of the bed frame, all the way around. Hit every crevice and don't forget the legs and casters too (if any).

Let everything sit to dry for at least 10 minutes. The alcohol spray will purge any mites that may be harboring in your bed. Now you can reassemble your bed.

This process may sound involved, but after you do it once or twice you'll find it only takes you a couple of minutes and goes a long way toward giving you a good night's sleep.

Once the bed is dry, open the plastic bag containing the set of freshly laundered bedding, and put it on the bed. Don't let the blanket or sheets touch the floor. Tuck the corners under the mattress. Now the bed is ready to use – but don't get in it yet!

Prepare Your Body for Bed

Every night without fail, you must take a bath or shower, immediately before going to bed. The moment you get out of the tub or shower, dry off with a clean towel, put on your sandals or flip flops, and *head straight to bed.*

Plan things so you don't need to walk around your home, or pause to do any tasks, or sit down anywhere. Just go *directly* from the bathroom to your bed. Step out of your sandals, and climb right into bed.

Again, any tasks such as getting a glass of water, watching the late show on TV, bolting the front door, saying your prayers, etc. should all be done BEFORE your bath or shower. Going directly to bed from the shower gives you the chance to climb into a clean bed without random mites jumping onto you. This gives you the best odds of a good night's sleep.

Shopping List #4

- Tinactin Antifungal Powder Spray or Lotramin Antifungal Powder Spray
- 12 rolls of paper towels (we like Bounty "Select a Size")
- Medicated body powder (optional)

Protect Your Entire Body

One of the most annoying behaviors of mites is their tendency to crawl around your private parts. This especially can happen at night. Mites migrate to the pelvic area, attracted by warmth and moisture. Mites also seem to prefer biting in skin creases, or wherever the skin is folded against itself. Perhaps, the tight spaces give them leverage to inflict deeper bites.

There are several ways to repel mites from these sensitive areas.

One defense is to apply medicated talcum powder after your bath, or better yet a powder spray, such as Tinactin Antifungal Powder Spray or Lotramin Antifungal Powder Spray. Some believe that fungus spores on the skin attract mites, so eliminating any trace of fungal infection helps.

We recommend after bathing and drying thoroughly, spray the crotch area with an antifungal powder spray. Do this after your morning shower, too.

This next tip may sound odd, but it's remarkably effective. After you make the bed each evening, place three clean paper towels by your pillow. Later, when you climb into bed, take the paper towels and fold one tightly into each of the three major skin creases of the groin area: the left upper inside thigh, the right upper inside thigh, and the buttocks. Just tuck them into those areas, and they should stay put on their own.

The towels not only absorb natural moisture, but also repel the mites from crawling in these areas. Be sure to tuck the paper towels fully into the skin creases for best results. We found this virtually eliminated bird mite activity in these sensitive areas.

It's best to not wear pajamas or a nightgown to bed. Fabric gives mites more places to hide. Sleeping naked may sound counterintuitive because your skin is fully exposed. But in reality, it's better than wearing any garments to bed. If you must wear something, make sure it contains 100% man-made fibers (polyester, rayon, etc.).

How Bird Mites Locate You

Mites have the uncanny ability to sense body heat, body chemistry, carbon dioxide exhaled, and perhaps other signals humans give off. The bugs use these signs to track you down in your home and jump onto you. Bird mites can crawl fairly fast and jump quite high, easily leaping from the floor up onto your bed. So you may feel one or more landing on you as you lay in bed.

If your home has a forced air system, it helps to run the system fan continuously at night. By circulating air around your home constantly, mites will find it more difficult to sense your exact location and zero in on you. We found this helpful.

In scientific experiments, bird mites were seen to travel up to 100 yards outdoors to reach a potential host. Indoors, they do the same. One way to discourage this is to keep the bedroom door closed at night, blocking the bottom of the door with a rolled up towel or blanket.

Chapter Ten: REPEL THE MITES

In researching bird mites, we learned of a number of ways to make the home less hospitable to them. We aren't convinced that every one of these ideas does much, but we share the research so you can be fully informed.

Shopping List #5

- Bag of Menthol Crystals
- Box of large black plastic garbage bags (for car seats)
- Several coffee mug warmers (AC powered)
- Food Grade Diatomaceous Earth (optional)
- Powder Duster for diatomaceous earth (optional)
- Power fogger machine (optional)

<u>Food grade Diatomaceous Earth</u>. If you try this, be certain you get FOOD GRADE, not the other type of diatomaceous earth commonly found at garden or home stores. The garden type is not healthy to use indoors.

<u>Duster Applicator</u>. Use this to apply a light coating of the diatomaceous earth wherever you don't want mites -- which in our case, meant everywhere in our home. We bought a 50 pound supply of diatomaceous earth, and ended up using maybe two pounds, which turned out to be plenty.

Supposedly, the microscopic diatomaceous earth particles are very jagged, and bird mites find this irritating. We dusted our entire place liberally for quite a while, but did not notice much improvement from this messy product. You may get better results. But if you don't appreciate having a layer of white dust on everything, you may not like this approach anyway.

The "Cides" There are products that are well-advertised as natural mite killers (let's nickname these products "the cides"). These are liquid sprays with different brand names and formulations.

We purchased several gallons of these, along with a costly power fogger, and treated our home. Our high hopes, based on the promises given, were dashed. While the stuff may work on other creatures, it did nothing to stop the bird mite infestation. It slowed it very slightly, for about 24 hours. Then the mites came back, and worse than ever.

In fact, we found these products seemed to aggravate the mites. Perhaps this was due to the moisture introduced by the stuff. As we keep repeating, moisture acts like fuel to bird mites. So we cannot recommend these products.

Menthol Crystals. This is a known bird mite repellent and we found this helpful.

First, purchase a supply of menthol crystals, along with one or two coffee mug warmer devices (the kind you plug in, to keep your java warm).

Place the mug warmer on a floor, in a room you wish to repel mites. Pour about a tablespoon of crystals in an old coffee mug or metal can (don't put crystals on the warmer itself).

Set the cup or can containing the crystals on the warmer, plug it in, and leave the room. In a short time, the menthol will start to vaporize, and the room will be filled with a totally overpowering mint aroma (sort of like menthol cough drops on steroids).

We'd sometimes place two or three of the menthol crystal setups in various rooms that had major mite issues, and leave them there for 6 to 8 hours.

Caution: the heat liquefies the menthol crystals. Avoid spilling the hot liquid.

Unfortunately, menthol vapor does not actually kill mites. It just drives them out of the area with vapors. We often used menthol in the living room during the day, so there would be fewer mites in that room at night, when we'd return home.

Another word of warning. We read about an apartment dweller who used the menthol crystals strategy. The mites ended up migrating to the next door neighbor's apartment! You do NOT want to inflict your mites on anyone else. So this approach is no good if you live in a multi-family dwelling.

Menthol crystals can be quite effective in an infested car, and we explain that process later.

"The Last Blast"

At one point when things were going really badly in our mite battle, we were truly desperate to find anything to slow the bugs down. Mites had become a major nuisance, in every room. Often they would crawl up onto the ceiling and drop down onto us. This was annoying, to say the least.

Since we already had purchased a power fogger (the "Tri-Jet Fogger 6208") for applying the "cide" products, we wondered what else we could spray with it. We had already learned that bird mites are resistant to pesticides and the "cide" products, so it was pointless to try those.

But a few substances seem to physically harm the bugs. One of these is ammonia. We hit upon the crazy idea of fogging the rooms with straight ammonia! This is risky, as ammonia fumes are very toxic. Breathing it is hazardous, as the fumes can really sting and burn the eyes, nose and throat.

If you do this, we recommend wearing goggles to protect your eyes.

A power fogger makes it possible to stand in the center of an infested room, flip the "on" switch, and rapidly blast a thick fog of ammonia into the far end of the room. You might feel like you're in the movie Ghostbusters.

While holding our breath, we'd quickly walk backwards toward the exit door, simultaneously fogging all four walls, the floor, and especially the ceiling. Once a room was fully blasted with ammonia fog (this only took about 10 seconds), we'd step outside the room and quickly shut the door. Even with this careful, planned approach, fumes were sometimes overpowering and hard to avoid.

NEVER attempt this with a hand sprayer. Only use an electric power fogger. The power nozzle will strongly blast the fog away from you. But with a hand sprayer, you'll be caught up in the middle of the toxic, choking ammonia cloud.

The good news is this blast of ammonia tactic did help quite a bit. It cut down the bird mite population by several notches, especially ridding them from the ceilings of our home. Clearly, it had stunned the mite population. Still, we only recommend this tactic for worst-case situations.

You may wonder if the ammonia fog damaged any of our home furnishings. Because we were careful not to soak any surfaces with ammonia, the fog cloud had no visible effect on anything. Painted surfaces, hardwood floors, framed pictures and wallpaper all seemed fine afterwords, in our experience. And the fumes dissipated fairly quickly.

Of course, we do not guarantee the ammonia fog won't affect your furnishings -- or your health. Use caution.

It is caustic stuff! We only present this "last blast" approach for informational purposes, along with all the other ideas we tried. As with all the techniques in this book -- you're on your own if you choose to try them.

While the fogger did cut down considerably on the bird mites for a while, it wasn't the "magic bullet" we were hoping for. A noticeable population of mites still survived the fogging. And like other things we tried, the fogging had less of an effect, the second and third times we did it.

Mites at the Workplace

If you go to a workplace each day, it's very possible you will transfer mites
to that location. If possible, find a way to apply the same effective techniques to your workplace, as at home. For example, keep a spray bottle of high strength alcohol on hand. Spray your chair and work area first thing in the

morning, and during the day as needed. This will help a lot.

Mites in a Vehicle

The car is another common location for infestation, if you're having a mite problem. Mites are transferred from your body and clothes to the interior of your vehicle. They can harbor in the seats, carpet and other spaces inside the typical car or truck. To combat this, cover the driver's seat with several black plastic trash bags to discourage mite movement, and seal the plastic bags with clear tape..

A vehicle is a good place to use menthol crystals (mentioned above). Mites are repelled from any location that has menthol vapors. They seem to hate these fumes. If it's summertime (or if you live in a warm climate), all you need to do is set a cup of menthol crystals on the floor of the car, on a sunny day. The interior heat will flood the car with menthol vapors, whichl totally permeate the interior, forcing the mites to exit. Be sure to leave one window open just slightly, to give the mites a clear place to exit. You will likely need to give an infested vehicle multiple treatments over time.

If there's limited sunshine in your area, or its cold outside, you can still treat your car with menthol. You'll need a cup warmer and a long extension cord. Drape the cord through one window of the car, which you left slightly open. Then plug in the cup warmer and set a mug on it containing a few teaspoons of menthol crystals.

Anytime you return to your car after a menthol treatment, you'll definitely want to open all the windows for a few minutes to air things out. The menthol fumes will at first be overpowering, making your eyes water. And you'll notice the fumes can linger, especially in hot summer weather. This is good. It keeps on repelling mites from your car interior.

Be careful not to spill the hot menthol liquid in your car. We suggest you place a large pie pan, or similar flat, metal container down first, and then place the cup heater on it. This way, if there's a spill the hot liquid menthol won't get on the interior.

One more important way to reduce mites in the car is to frequently go over the interior with a heavy duty vacuum. We used a shop vac on the carpeting, seats, dashboard, door panels, rear deck, and headliner, about once a week. If you don't own a heavy duty vacuum, your local car wash probably has a coin-operated one.

A final suggestion for the car, if your vehicle has fabric floor mats. Replace them with solid rubber mats. Store away the fabric mats in sealed trash bags, for the time being.

You can even apply carpet protection film (see Chapter Six) to your car's carpeted floor, as we did, to minimize the areas in the vehicle where mites can congregate.

Chapter Eleven: HOST NO MORE

Now let's talk about one more very important part of winning the battle: making YOU less attractive as a host to bird mite parasites.

If you've been reading along so far, you'll recall that natural fibers are a very attractive environment for bird mites. Thus our recommendation to store away or seal up the rugs and other furnishings, along with cotton and wool clothes, etc. The reason is simple. In nature, bird mites attach themselves to winged creatures by grabbing onto the feathers and natural fiber shafts of the birds. They also like to burrow in and lay their eggs in this natural fiber environment.

Well, guess what – the mites will act the very same way with you!

Of course, humans don't have feathers, but we do have hair. Most of us have hair all over our bodies, although on some areas of the skin, it may be very fine and nearly invisible. Body hair is no doubt one big reason bird mites find humans attractive as hosts. All that body hair gives bird mites an inviting, familiar home.

Never before have we had any reason to shave every square inch of skin. But now we were open to trying *anything* to help eliminate the mite infestation.

Interestingly, removing body hair never crossed our mind, until the day we read about a man whose entire family was infested with *lice*. Lice are tiny parasites that harbor themselves in the scalp. Commonly, kids catch lice from other school children, and the youngsters spread the parasites to others, sometimes family members.

The lice removal process involves shampooing the hair with a pesticide-based product, along with tedious manual removal of tiny eggs (nits) from the hair, using a special fine-tooth comb.

This particular news story said that rather than deal with the lice problem, this man decided that he and his entire family would simply shave their heads! Problem solved. They also became the talk of the town.

An Obvious Idea

Reading this amusing story gave me an idea. I quickly decided to make it tougher for mites to harbor themselves on me, by shaving every single part of my skin!

You may not realize how much hair is on your body until you try this.

Be warned, if you're male and do a full body shave in the shower, all that hair may end up clogging the drain. And it might take you a while to shave it all off the first time, too.

Most women are used to shaving their legs and underarms. But for both men and women, it may feel awkward shaving your entire body -- arms, chest, back, and so on. If you've never before shaved your genital area, that takes special care. In our case, once all the shaving was done -- we noticed an immediate drop in mite activity on our bodies!

You might not bother shaving some areas such as your forearms, because you think the hair growth is minimal there. You may notice the mites remain active in those areas. So be sure to carefully shave every square inch of your skin. It can really make a difference.

A Close Shave

At first, it will be time-consuming to add body shaving to your list every day. But soon the shaving will become faster and easier, as you get used to it.

You may also get a few nicks and scrapes early on, due to unfamiliarity with body shaving. But those are nothing, compared to the benefit of getting rid of the body hair.

Many men have noticeable hair on their back. Most women do too, to a lesser degree. It can be difficult to shave your own back, unless you have a spouse to help -

- or a product designed for this purpose. Luckily, a long-handled, battery operated shaver is made just for this purpose. It's called the Mangroomer and it makes shaving the back much easier.

Body hair grows quickly. Mites seem to gravitate to it. You may find it helpful to keep a disposable razor handy at all times. When you feel a mite crawling on you, give a few quick swipes with the dry blade to remove the mite, along with any peach fuzz in that area.

If you believe there's no hair of any kind growing on your body, try examining your skin in very bright light (such as direct sunlight). Look closely at the surface of your skin (such as your forearm). You will be surprised at how much hair there actually is. Bird mites find even the finest, thinnest hair to be a welcome environment.

Get a Haircut

After shaving my body, I continued to have problems with bird mites crawling on my scalp. With no hair on the body, the little buggers naturally go for the hair on the head. Most people reading this will draw the line at adopting the "bald look" (although some might choose to go that route).

This is a helpful compromise that we tried instead. We had the stylist give us a short buzz cut. We hoped it would help, and sure enough, it did. It really reduced the crawling bird mites on the scalp. Yes, there was still a little mite activity from time to time, but noticeably less than before.

Here's what we recommend. First, give full body shaving a try. Get your entire body "clean as a baby's bottom".

And for both men and women, consider getting a buzz cut. This will make a big difference in reducing the mites on your scalp. Remember, your hair will grow back again. This isn't a permanent change.

Shopping List #6

- Nit-Free Mousse for the hair
- Selsun Blue medicated shampoo
- Dr. Bronner's Peppermint Soap
- Epsom Salts
- Curel "Itch Defense" lotion or Lubriderm "Sensitive" lotion
- Vicks Vap-O-Rub
- Eurax cream (optional)

Bust that Protein Glue

Another hair-related product may prove helpful to you, as it did for us. We had learned that when mites lay their eggs, they use a protein "glue" to attach the microscopic eggs to the host, until they hatch. Then the next generation of mites starts crawling around on your body.

In our research we learned of a hair product that is used to eliminate lice. It's called Nit-Free Mousse. This is not a pesticide. It's an enzyme that simply dissolves the protein that glues the eggs (nits) to the hair.

While lice are completely different creatures from mites, we decided to try it anyway. Our thought was it might help get rid of the bird mite eggs that were glued to our hair and scalp, since mites also use protein glue. The product is non-toxic, and available over the counter at most drug stores or Amazon.com.

This liquid enzyme only attacks the protein holding the eggs in place. (By the way, this company makes a number of products under the "Nit-Free" brand – be sure to get the <u>mousse</u>, which comes in a foam applicator bottle.)

To use it, first wash and rinse your hair, using any shampoo. Then apply enough "puffs" of the Nit-Free mousse foam to coat your hair (if you have a buzz cut, you won't need much). Avoid the eyes. Massage the foam into the scalp and then let it sit there and work for about 5 minutes, to dissolve the mite protein glue. Then *without rinsing,* do a second treatment with the mousse, again letting it work for 5 minutes. Now -- rinse well. An added benefit you'll quickly notice: your hair will be absolutely squeaky clean after this treatment.

You can use the enzyme treatment as often as you wish We sometimes did it twice a day. It was very helpful in keeping our hair free of crawling mites, presumably because it washed away the eggs in our hair, sending them down the drain before they could hatch.

More Hair Products

There are anti-mite websites which suggest a multitude of hair products. We won't repeat them all here, other than the ones that actually seemed to help.

One product we used early on was Denorex Therapeutic (Coal Tar) shampoo. Whew, this is strong stuff. It's not something we could use very often, because it was so overpowering. But it did seem to have a repellent effect.

Another we used more often was Selsun Blue Medicated Shampoo, in the red and blue bottle (there are other Selsun Blue products, but this is their strongest). It's not quite as irritating as Denorex, so for a time we used it daily. It seemed to help. The shampoo can also be used as body wash.

Dr. Bronner's Peppermint Liquid Soap is found at natural food stores such as Whole Foods. Bird mites are repelled by strong aromatic oils such as menthol. This product is very minty! We used it as a body wash and shampoo, and found it fairly effective at repelling mites.

Bath and Shower Tips

During our mite infestation, we tried many bath and shower products. Here's one that really helped us.

On those days when we just couldn't seem to get free of aggressive mites, we would find blessed relief in a hot bath, with a cup of Epsom salts dissolved in the water. This was temporary relief, sometimes the only time in the entire day when we would not feel mites crawling. Sometimes we'd add bubble bath or moisturizer to the bath water just for variety. However, once the Epsom salt bath was over, and we'd return to our activities, the mites would soon be back.

Keep in mind, bird mites can withstand temperatures below freezing and over 125 degrees. So bathing in very hot water, even a strong salt solution, isn't going to kill mites. The Epsom salt bath does seem to slow their activity, though.

Sometimes, we would feel a mite biting hard DURING a bath or shower, often on our legs, feet, or toes. We think it was a final attack before a floating mite headed down the drain.

Some bath additives we tried included tea tree oil, eucalyptus oil, spearmint oil, peppermint oil, Batherapy

Sport, Borax powder (NOT recommended, our borax bath caused some dizziness). We even tried bathing in a mild bleach solution. None of these made much difference at all.

We also read about a lime sulfur pet-dip product (used for giving a flea-infested pet a bath). Somebody said it could be used by mite-infested humans, as well. We tried the product. It smelled awful and did nothing to stop the mites.

Skin Hygiene

Every day without fail, we applied unscented moisturizing skin cream all over, after every bath or shower. This was very helpful in minimizing irritation and rashes from the mite bites, while greatly reducing itchiness.

The two best products for this we found were Curel "Itch Defense" lotion, and Lubriderm "Sensitive" 100% fragrance-free lotion. Both cut down on the itchy skin problems considerably.

Still More Skin Products

There is a prescription cream we were able to order via the Internet at one point. It is both an anti-itch medication and an anti-scabies treatment. The active ingredient is crotamiton. Eurax is the product brand name. It actually gave total itch relief, and freedom from crawling, from head to toe for 24 hours when we used it. Unfortunately, it was costly, difficult to apply, and time-consuming to obtain. It did help during the short time we used it, but for obvious reasons, was not a long term solution. Also it was far less effective, the second time we tried it.

Varying our skin treatments seemed to keep the mites confused, at least. We had momentary success using anti perspirants, muscle "heat" creams, and Sulfur 8 Cream. We even rubbed our skin with fabric softener sheets, and a strong mouthwash like Listerine. All had momentary effect, but nothing worked long term.

To keep mites off toes and feet (a nightly nuisance), we regularly applied Vicks Vapo-Rub to the feet and toes, every night after climbing into bed.

We'd also apply it around the nose, ears and mouth, to discourage mites from entering those openings during the night. We previously mentioned the *paper towel defense* which was a big help for the pelvic area, while Vicks helped protect facial openings and the feet. A side benefit to applying Vicks to the toes every night -- toenails will look more healthy than ever before.

We also kept a spray bottle of high strength alcohol by the bed at all times. It was very helpful to blast on the body when we'd feel mites moving.

A mechanical way to remove mites from the skin is with an adhesive lint roller. You roll the sticky tape over the skin when you feel movement and activity. You need to change the roll to a fresh adhesive surface fairly often. Doing this was somewhat helpful, but not as effective as using the alcohol spray.

Dietary Recommendations

As the saying goes, you are what you eat. It's highly possible that mites are more or less attracted to you, based upon the foods you regularly eat. If you often eat a high carbohydrate diet with plenty of starch and sugar, this can make mites more aggressive.

Let's face it, nearly every creature is attracted to sugar, just as humans are. So we suggest cutting down on the carbs and sugary drinks and desserts, to reduce mite activity. If your body chemistry contains lower metabolic byproducts of sugar, you will be "less tasty" to biting bird mites.

Chapter Twelve: ELIMINATE THEM ALL

Summarizing the previous recommendations, the way to total mite elimination first requires these critical steps to reduce and weaken the population:

- Use a clothes washing machine with a steam cycle
- Shave all body hair, consider a buzz cut for your head
- Regularly wash scalp with enzyme product
- Frequently vacuum house and car, eliminate all clutter
- Seal all fabric furnishings in plastic (rugs/curtains/bedding)
- Wear clothes/shoes of polyester/nylon -- no cotton/wool
- Treat vehicle with menthol crystals
- Lower humidity level at home

All these steps made a noticeable difference by weakening the bird mite population. But they did not fully solve the problem. Some days were better, some worse. Still, the infestation went on.

The initial scale of our mite invasion meant the army of parasites were settled into our home for the long term. Short of a miracle breakthrough, some mites would keep surviving, generation after generation. Despite our best efforts, the pests kept evolving and adapting, and their population remained active.

So we bit the bullet and decided we had to find a second place to live. We would vacate our first home, until all the mites in it were dead.

Our budget was limited. We found a rental advisor and told her we needed an unfurnished place, ideally with tile or stone floors, "due to allergies". In just one day, she found a place we liked. We signed a lease and set the move-in date with the landlord.

We began making preparations to stay away from home, for at least *six months*. Without a host to feed upon, no mites can survive for six months.

To prepare for the move, we first collected all important papers and other items we might need. All these items were sealed in plastic bags. We also arranged to have the mail forwarded to our rental place by the post office.

However, we did not want to bring any clothes or even a suitcase from our home to the new place. We knew this would bring many mites to the new place.

This is how we handled the transition to the new place.

On the day of our move, we closed up our home, locked the door, and drove to Wal-Mart. There we bought new clothes, athletic shoes, bedding and towels, toiletries, and a new suitcase. All items remained in the plastic bags from the store. Now we drove to the new apartment.

Immediately upon arrival, we stripped. We put every stitch of the clothes we were wearing into a trash bag, double bagged it, and tossed it in the garbage. We jumped into the shower, scrubbing body and hair, and using the enzyme product. We dried off with a brand new towel, and put on a new set of clothes. Then we called the mattress store to deliver a new bed.

A Spartan Life

In the new home, we lived a spartan life over the next six months. Things were simple, with minimal furniture. We just had some metal folding chairs, a laptop computer, a small dining table, and a twin bed. We covered the bed with plastic film (as explained previously). And we continued to follow all the same daily home cleaning rituals and body hygiene rituals as we had done back at our home.

It was so great to be out of our home, away from the endless mite infestation! From day one, we slept better each night in the new place.

About that same time, though our vehicle was not badly infested, we decided to trade it in for another used car. We were making a clean break from the past.

Despite all the planning, a few mites naturally survived the trip to the new rental apartment. We still got an occasional bite or felt a random crawling sensation. However, the new place had tile floors and limited furnishings. It was a harsh environment for the remaining bird mites. Plus, there was no established mite population living in all the cracks and crevices, as at our home.

Thanks to our ongoing hygiene and cleansing procedures (as outlined in past chapters), we noticed a gradual lessening of mites.

Then one day, we suddenly realized they were completely gone. No more bites or crawling at all. What a blessing!

We hesitated to celebrate, however. We figured it was just a lull in the action. But as the weeks turned into months, we realized the bird mites were finally out of our life.

Since the infestation first began, it had taken a toll on us for nearly a year. There had been much suffering and lots of experimentation, and significant expense. And we should add, prayer and determination. But the final result was success.

The Day We Returned Home

Then came the fateful day when it was time to leave the rental and return to our old home. Would there still be active mites in the old place? Since we moved out, we'd drive by the house periodically to make sure everything looked OK from the outside. But we hadn't dared go inside or even go near the front door, until today. It had been a full six months since we closed up and vacated the place.

With great trepidation, we unlocked the front door and stepped inside. We stood in the hallway, waiting to feel if mites would jump on us, eagerly bite and attack, as we'd felt so many times before. But this time, there was nothing. The front hallway was completely dead.

Encouraged, we walked through every room, standing for a while in each space. It felt strange to be back in the place after so long. But it was even stranger to not find any mites waiting for us. They had either died off or gone elsewhere!

In fact we suspect some vacated the place for the great outdoors, after it became clear that their human meal ticket had gone away. This is the same behavior bird mites follow when a bird abandons an infested nest. The remaining mites must go find a new host, or else they starve to death. That's how the mites first found us, migrating from a dead robin into our home, where they found a new (human) host.

Possibly, the mites moved out of our home to find wild birds or other creatures on the outside.

No Mites At All

As afternoon turned to evening, it was soon bedtime.

We felt more trepidation as we went to bed. But again, no mites at all. Nothing at all bothered us.

Obviously that six month hiatus was just what it took for the entire mite population to either die away or depart. And since our body was now mite-free, there weren't any new mites for us to introduce to the home environment.

Our desire for caution convinced us to keep rugs, clothes, and other fabric items sealed in their plastic cocoons for another six months. We also kept up the house cleaning and body hygiene rituals, which by then, were deeply ingrained habits (we still follow some of those rituals today to keep clean).

Months later, when we finally opened the plastic bags and unsealed the rugs, there was no mite activity whatsoever. And it felt great to suddenly get our favorite cotton and wool clothes back again, and to sleep on cotton sheets once more.

Alternative Solution?

As you have read here, the bird mite situation in our home improved over time as we learned which strategies worked and which didn't, and we began to apply those ideas to our living conditions.

Despite that, we could never break free and eliminate all bird mites until we took the bold step of leaving home for six months. We needed a temporary home with tile floors and very limited furnishings to help stop the endless cycle of parasite reproduction in our home.

Had we simply moved to a new place, without following the initial mite elimination steps (see bullet points at the beginning of this chapter), we doubt it would have ended the problem. We would have just brought all the mites with us, to the new place.

Weaken Them First

So we are convinced that the preliminary steps were critical, to greatly weaken the mite population. Then when we moved to a new place, it was far easier to kill the remaining population off completely.

Luckily, thanks to this book you now know what works and what doesn't. You can avoid all the trial and error, and simply apply the proven formulas we discovered.

Yes, it's a lot of work. Yes, your life will be disrupted. But you will get through it and come out fine on the other side.

You may be wondering something right now: what to do if your budget is severely limited, and moving to a second temporary home isn't possible?
Well, if you have a relatively light infestation of mites, then the recommended steps at the beginning of the

chapter may be all you need. That might completely take care of the problem.

But if those steps do not eliminate all the mites, then the "killing blow" of a six month move from home may be necessary.

More Ideas To Consider

Here are some other ideas to think about, if you have a very limited budget:

1) Split your existing home in two. In other words, move out of half of your home, completely sealing up the first half so that every crack and crevice is closed off from the other half. Live in the other section for six months, which will allow the mites to completely die off in the first half of your home. Then, very carefully and quickly reserve the process – move into the mite-free zone, sealing off the still infested half of your home. This will give you a reasonable chance of eliminating the mites in your life once and for all.

2) Find a foreclosure. Sometimes, home mortgage holders fail to make their payments, and homes are foreclosed upon. This means that a number of homes in any part of the country sit vacant. There may be an empty, foreclosed home available to rent for six months at very low cost – possibly, just in exchange for upkeep and maintenance. Obviously, you shouldn't tell a realtor about your bird mite problem. Instead, you might say

your home needs improvements, which will take six months. And you need a very affordable place to stay, during that period of time. Is there an empty or foreclosed home available for short-term lease (preferably with tile or stone floors)?

These are just a few ideas. There may be other ways to solve the dilemma of finding a second home for six months.

Never Give Up

Where there's a will, there's a way. Whatever you do, don't give up or resign yourself to endless suffering. Explore every option. Maintain your regular cleaning routines for home and body. Be bold and sport a buzz cut for a while, whether you're male or female!

Something we soon realized during our ordeal: whenever we'd feel down or depressed and plunk ourselves down in front of a screen for hours at a time, or just try to forget, nothing improved. In fact, things just got worse. Sitting motionless in the evening just made the mites more relentless.

But when we got up and kept moving, took action and tried new things, the situation gradually improved (although there were good and bad days).

Remember that saying "God doesn't give us anything we can't handle". We learned a lot about ourselves, and about inner strength and persistence, during the mite invasion. At times it was sad and lonely, and that feeling is perfectly human. But we never gave up the fight. By not giving up, we achieved victory.

It has been years since our bird mite infestation first began and ended. While it was a mental ordeal to go back and reconstruct all that we went through, we hope these strategies are helpful to you.

We have now fulfilled a promise we made to ourselves, to share what we learned during our ordeal, with others who are dealing with a bird mite infestation.

What promise can you make to yourself? What will you do for yourself and for others, once your mite problem is solved? Have the vision of a positive end goal. That is something that kept us moving forward with hope, in the most difficult hours.

Our hopes and best wishes go out to you and your family, for complete and everlasting mite eradication.

Appendix

Here are excerpts of research studies referencing the **Northern Avian Mite** (bird mite or fowl mite). These brief excerpts are presented under section 107 of the Copyright Act of 1976, in which allowance is made for "fair use" including education and research.

1. <u>Fowl Mites</u> by A.L. Antonelli, Washington State Univ. Ext. Entomologist. Updated May 2003.

"Two species of fowl mites, the Northern fowl mite, *Ornithonyssus sylviarum* (Fig. 1), and the chicken mite, *Dermanyssus gallinae*, may attack humans when the right circumstances prevail....Household infestations can result when chicken roosts or wild bird nests...are in close proximity to the home. The bite of the chicken mite can be particularly painful and irritating. These mites are extremely small....Invariably, when household mite infestations are determined...the pest turns out to be one of these fowl mites."

2. <u>Northern Fowl Mite Dermatitis</u> by Huynh Congly, MSc. Provincial Laboratories, Saskatchewan Department of Health. April 1985.

"*O. sylviarum* is a common ecto-parasite of a variety of wild and domestic birds, including swallows, robins, sparrows and chickens. It occurs in all temperate and some tropical regions. Adult mites are vicious, blood-sucking, nonburrowing parasites that spend most of their life on the body of the bird host....The northern fowl mite may attack a human when its normal host is not available."

3. Acaricide [pesticide] Resistance in Northern Fowl Mite (*Ornithonyssus sylviarum*) Populations on Caged Layer Operations in So. California by B. A. Mullens, et. al. Dept. of Entomology & U. of California Coop. Ext., U. of Cal. Oct. 2004.

"The northern fowl mite, *O. sylviarum*...is considered to be the most important ectoparasite of poultry in North America..... Mites complete the entire life cycle on the host...while feeding on blood, and the generation interval is only 5 to 12 days....populations thus can become very high....To our knowledge this is the first documentation of widespread and extreme resistance to permethrin [pesticide]...in northern fowl mite populations...."

4. Mites Affecting Humans by Illinois Department of Health. Undated.

"Mites that normally infest birds also bite people. The northern fowl mite (*O. sylviarum*) and chicken mite (*Dermanyssus gallinae*) primarily infest chickens, but also pigeons, starlings and sparrows."

5. <u>Chronic Pruritis: An Uncommon Cause</u> by Aditya K. Gupta, MD; et. al. The Medical Center, Ann Arbor. Undated.

"Dermatosis in humans caused by avian mites...may result from the mites that infest chickens, ducks, pigeons, canaries, sparrows, starlings, robins, and tiger finches....species include *O. sylviarum* (northern fowl mite) and *O. bursa* (tropical fowl mite)."

6. <u>Northern Fowl Mite</u> by P. E. Kaufman, et. al. Entomology & Nematology Dept. Fla. Coop. Ext. Service, Institute of Food and Agri. Sciences, U. of Florida. July 2009.

"The northern fowl mite...is widely distributed... throughout many of the temperate regions of the world parasitizing domestic fowl and wild birds....Also of considerable importance, the mites will bite man... causing itching and irritation to the skin....Adult female mites take a blood meal and complete egg-laying in 2 days....The complete life cycle from egg to egg-laying female can take place in 5-7 days or longer depending on temperature and humidity. Adult mites spend most of their lives on the host, but will also wander to the eggs or rafters [ceiling]."

Notes

Notes